First Aid/Emergencies

(A Complete Patient Care Guide)

Third Edition

First Aid/Emergencies

(A Complete Patient Care Guide)

Third Edition

V.K. Jain
Banswara
Rajasthan

PEEPEE
PUBLISHERS AND DISTRIBUTORS (P) LTD.

First Aid/Emergencies
(A Complete Patient Care Guide)

Published by
Pawaninder P. Vij

Peepee Publishers and Distributors (P) Ltd.
Head Office: 160, Shakti Vihar, Pitam Pura
Delhi-110 034 (India)

Correspondence Address:

7/31, Ansari Road, Daryaganj
Post Box-7243, New Delhi-110 002 (India)

Ph: 65195868, 23246245, 9811156083

e-mail: peepee160@yahoo.co.in

e-mail: peepee160@rediffmail.com

e-mail: peepee160@gmail.com

www.peepeepub.com

First Edition: **2004**

Third Edition: **2010**

ISBN: 81-8445-089-3

Printed at
Lordson, C-5/19, Rana Pratap Bagh, Delhi-110 007

Preface to the Third Edition

Emergency Medicine is the most demanding field in medicine. It needs an urgent action coming from a thoughtful and decision making mind. Emergency Medicine is a highly skilled area of medicine. This book is intended for the medical practitioners, nurses as well as for a layman. I have tried to include the FIRST AID for the commonly encountered emergency situations in the day-to-day life. My special thanks to Dr. Charu Mittal for contributing chapter on Labor Pain and Delivery. I hope you will acknowledge my efforts and will encourage me to improve my writings in future.

V.K. Jain

Contents

Chapter 1

Allergies

Allergic reactions are caused by a hypersensitive immune system that reacts when it is exposed to a usually harmless substance. For example, if you're allergic to peanuts and you eat a substance that has peanut extract in it your body will react against this harmless substance as though it were a bacterium, virus, or other harmful toxin. Often the exposure to an allergen needs only to be slight for a reaction to occur, and sometimes a reaction may not occur for several hours.

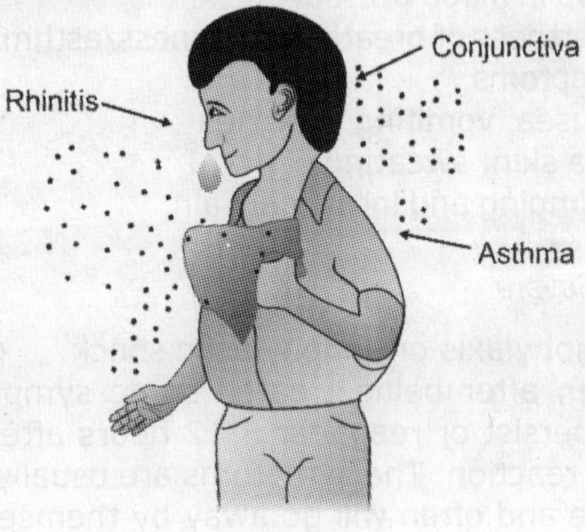

Some Common Allergens Are

Food: Nuts, shellfish, egg, wheat, beans, citrus, milk, additives Medicines: penicillin, ibuprofen, aspirin, latex (gloves, condoms etc). *Plants & animals:* Pet dander, poison ivy, insect stings/bites, pollen, grass, dust.

Symptoms

Mild Reactions (most common)

- Itching
- Flushed skin
- Hives
- Coughing, sneezing
- Headaches
- Asthma like symptoms (wheezing, coughing, shortness of breath)
- Red or watery eyes.

More Severe Reactions

- Intense hives
- Intense itching
- Swelling of the face, eyes, tongue, throat
- Difficulty swallowing (often because of swelling)
- Increased heart rate
- Drop in blood pressure
- Shortness of breath, hoarseness/asthma like symptoms
- Nausea, vomiting, diarrhea
- Pale skin, sweating
- Cramping and intestinal pain.

Most Severe

- Anaphylaxis or anaphylactic shock.

Even after being treated some symptoms may persist or reappear 8-12 hours after the initial reaction. The symptoms are usually less severe and often will go away by themselves. Some symptoms, such as hives, will appear and disappear over 4-6 hours, even if the person is no longer being exposed to the allergen. Hives may last for several days or even weeks, so over the counter antihistamines, like Benadryl, can be used to treat hives.

Treatment

One of the easiest ways to prevent allergic reactions is to avoid the substances that cause the reactions. If you leave your children in the care of a babysitter it is important to let them know if the child has any allergies and what to do if a reaction occurs.

If a reaction does occur most (mild, and some more serious reactions) can be treated with antihistamines, like Benadryl. These stop the asthma like reactions, and cold like symptoms. Those with ***asthma*** should be especially careful if they are highly allergic to a substance.

If the reaction takes place on the skin use ice wrapped in a towel, cool oatmeal baths, and hydrocortisone cream to lessen the itching and swelling. If these things don't help, call your doctor. With things like poison ivy, you should wash everything the person who touched the plant has touched to avoid spreading it further and causing more reactions among them or other people. Wash everything, skin, hair, clothing, toys, countertops, and even pets.

If you think the reaction may be due to a medication the child has taken, immediately stop treatment and contact a doctor.

Even mild reactions should be treated quickly, because if they go untreated the reaction may jump from a mild to a serious reaction in a short amount of time. In more severe cases ***CPR*** and oxygen may need to be administered.

For some people it is very hard to avoid the substance they are allergic to. For these people a more expensive, but more permanent option is available. Immunotherapy, or allergy shots, is small doses of the allergen that are given to the patient and increased over time in order to develop an immunity to the allergen. They are almost 100% effective but usually require at least 5 years of monthly (in some cases weekly) shots.

For those who are very allergic to a substance often only a slight encounter with an allergen will send them into a potentially fatal reaction known as anaphylaxis, or anaphylactic

shock. In these cases, time is very important and epinephrine (Epipen) must be administered. Unless you are trained, do not administer the shot, call for help instead.

House Dust Allergy

House dust allergy is common even in clean homes. House dust is a major cause of year-round runny or stuffy nose, itchy, watery eyes and sneezing for allergy sufferers. Dust can also make people with asthma experience wheezing, coughing and shortness of breath.

Why Does House Dust Cause Allergic Reactions?

House dust is a mixture of many substances. Its content varies from home to home, depending on the type of furniture, building materials, presence of pets, moisture and other factors. A speck of dust may contain fabric fibers, human skin particles, animal dander, microscopic creatures called mites, bacteria, parts of cockroaches, mold spores, food particles and other debris. Of these, animal dander, house dust mites and cockroaches are the most common culprits. A person may be allergic to one or more of these substances, and, if exposed to the dust, will have an allergic reaction.

Is Dust Allergy a Sign of a Dirty House?

No. A dirty house can make a house dust allergy problem worse, however. Normal housekeeping procedures may not be enough to get rid of house dust allergy symptoms. This is because many of the substances in dust cannot be removed by normal cleaning procedures. For example, no matter how vigorously you dust or vacuum, you will not reduce the number of dust mites present deep within carpeting, pillows and mattresses. Vigorous cleaning methods can put more dust into the air making symptoms worse.

What are Dust Mites?

Tiny microscopic creatures called dust mites are an important cause of allergic reactions to house dust. They belong to the family of eight-legged creatures called arachnids. This family also includes spiders, chiggers and ticks. Dust mites are hardy creatures that live well and multiply easily in warm, humid places. They prefer temperatures at or above 70 degrees Fahrenheit with a relative humidity of 75 percent to 80 percent and die when the humidity falls below 40 percent to 50 percent. They are rarely found in dry climates.

As many as 10 percent of the general population and 90 percent of people with allergic asthma are sensitive to dust mites. Recent studies in the United States suggest that at least 45 percent of young people with asthma are allergic to dust mites.

People who are allergic to dust mites react to proteins in the bodies and feces of the mites. These fecal particles are found in the highest concentrations in pillows, mattresses, carpeting and upholstered furniture. They float into the air when anyone vacuums, walks on a carpet or disturbs bedding, but settle out of the air once the disturbance is over. Dust mite-allergic people who inhale these particles frequently experience allergy symptoms. In fact, a dust mite allergic patient who sleeps for eight hours every night spends one third of his life with his nose in direct contact with a pillow loaded with dust mite particles!

There may be many as 19,000 dust mites in one gram of dust, but usually between 100 to 500 mites live in each gram. (A gram is about the weight of a paper clip.) Each mite produces about 10 to 20 waste particles per day and lives for 30 days. Egg-laying females can add 25 to 30 new mites to the population during their lifetime.

Mites eat particles of skin and dander, so they thrive in places where there are people.

Dust mites don't bite, cannot spread diseases and usually do not live on people. They are harmful only to people who become allergic to them. While usual household insecticides have no effect on dust mites, there are ways to reduce exposure to dust mites in the home.

Why is Mold Present in House Dust?

Molds are commonly found in outdoor air. However, any house can develop a mold problem given the right conditions. You might not see it growing on the walls, but it may still be present in your home. Molds require two factors to grow indoors: (1) free moisture that can occur in the form of relative humidity above 50 percent, leakage from pipes or foundations, or any ongoing source of water; and (2) something to grow on. Molds particularly like to grow on wallboard, wood or fabrics, but will grow virtually any place if they are given a chance.

Molds spread by producing spores that can become airborne. These spores end up in house dust where they grow. Dust from mold-contaminated houses can cause allergy symptoms if a mold-sensitive person inhales it.

Does House Dust Contain Cockroaches?

As unappealing as it seems, some houses do have dust that contains parts of cockroaches. This is most common in older, multifamily housing. Allergic individuals, particularly those with asthma, will tend to have increased symptoms when they go into such houses. Cockroaches require food and moisture to survive, so eliminating sources of each can help reduce exposure.

Is House Dust Allergy Seasonal?

Dust mite populations tend to peak in April and October, and their allergen levels stay high through December. Mite allergen levels are lowest in late spring. Some dust mite-sensitive people report that their symptoms get worse during the winter. That's because mite fecal particles and pieces of dead mites, both of which trigger dust mite allergy, are still present. Mold levels tend to peak during the summer months depending on where you live since some tropical areas have molds year-round. There is also evidence that cockroaches have a seasonal pattern, peaking in the late summer.

Forced-air heating systems tend to blow dust particles into the air. As they dry out over time, even more of the particles become airborne. This does not account for the seasonal pattern, however, since air blows through the same ducts during the summer when air conditioning is used. People may have fewer symptoms from house-dust exposure during the summer because they spend more time outdoors.

How Do I know if I have House Dust Allergy?

If you think you may have an allergy to house dust, consult an allergist-immunologist. To pinpoint the cause of your symptoms, the allergist may ask questions about your work and home environments, eating habits, family medical history, frequency and severity of symptoms, exposure to pets and a variety of other questions. Your allergist may test you for allergy by doing skin tests, which involves pricking the skin or injecting it with different allergens and observing for a reaction. A positive reaction (a raised welt with redness around it) may indicate that you are allergic to that allergen. Occasionally, your allergist may order a blood test instead of the skin test to confirm the diagnosis of allergy.

What Can I Do to Relieve House Dust Allergy Symptoms?

The three basic treatments for dust mite allergy are:

- Dust mite avoidance
- Prescription medications
- Allergy shots (immunotherapy).

House dust avoidance works best to relieve symptoms.

How Do I Avoid House Dust?

Environmental control of house dust exposure is best done if you know what allergens present in your home's dust are causing the problem. Dust mites can be difficult to remove completely from your home. However, you can follow certain anti-mite procedures that will reduce mite populations and your exposure to them, thereby reducing your symptoms. Some of these procedures are difficult, and you may not need to do them all. Ask your allergist which ones will be most helpful for your situation.

Pay Special Attention to Bedrooms

On average, people spend one-third of their lives in the bedroom. Studies have shown that, of all the rooms in the home, the bedroom often contains the most dust mites. Concentrate efforts in the bedroom of the dust-sensitive person.

- Select non-allergic, washable bedding materials. Rather than pillows stuffed with feathers, down, kapok or foam rubber, use pillows stuffed with synthetic materials. Get special casings (plastic or rubberized fabric) that zip around mattresses, box springs and pillows. These limit your exposure to dust mite particles. Avoid bulky comforters and chenille bedspreads. Use washable blankets and spreads, and wash all bedding (including pillows without cases) every week to 10 days, using hot water.
- If possible, install a room air conditioner and dehumidifier in the bedroom if the home does not have central air-conditioning. Lowering humidity reduces the number of mites, molds

and cockroaches. Avoid using vaporizers or humidifiers.

- Place a filter made of cheesecloth under the faceplate of the bedroom-heating vent to help prevent circulation of dust into the bedroom air and change it frequently.
- Hang clothes in a closet and keep the closet door closed, or put them into dresser drawers.
- Get rid of stuffed animals or use washable ones.
- Never allow pets in the bedroom.

Reduce Surface Dust

- Clean your home thoroughly on a regular basis (particularly the bedrooms). Vacuum frequently and dust with a damp or oiled cloth. Ideally, someone other than the dust-sensitive person should clean, but if this is impossible, wear a mask. Vacuuming can raise a cloud of dust. Special vacuum cleaner bags for trapping dust are available, and for some patients a central vacuum system may be advisable. You physician may also suggest use of a HEPA (High Efficiency Particulate Arresting) air filtered vacuum. These expensive units are not necessary for all patients.
- You may need to remove carpeting, especially in the bedroom. Carpeting is a breeding ground for dust mites. If you must have carpeting, select a type with low pile. Scatter rugs that can be washed each week are a better alternative. Wood floors, seamless vinyl or linoleum floor coverings are best because they can be cleaned easily and thoroughly, and mites don't like to live on uncarpeted floors.
- You may need to remove from your home any items that tend to collect or hold dust and replace them with easy-to-clean items. Use wooden, leather or plastic-covered sofas and chairs instead of upholstered furniture. Select closed bookcases and curio cabinets

instead of open shelves. Books and knick-knacks are dust collectors. Use washable curtains or window shades instead of Venetian blinds and heavy draperies. Choose furniture with simple, clean designs instead of ornately carved pieces. Select easily cleaned decorations instead of dried-flower arrangements, wall hangings and straw baskets.

Reduce Dust in the Air

- Use air-conditioning to keep inside humidity at 50 percent or lower to slow the growth of dust mites and molds during warm weather months. An inexpensive hygrometer will help you monitor humidity.
- Change or clean air-conditioner and furnace filters often. In some cases, your physician may recommend using a HEPA cleaner on your heating system or a portable HEPA filter unit in your bedroom. The portable units are efficient at cleaning air in their immediate vicinity, but are of limited use in large rooms. They have not been shown to be useful for patients with dust mite allergy, since the dust mite particles are not airborne.

What Products are Available to Get Rid of Dust Mites?

Certain chemicals kill dust mites or inactivate dust mite allergens. They are expensive, and some products can be respiratory irritants for some people. In general, their use is reserved for situations when the above measures have been tried and have failed.

Tannic acid destroys mite allergens but does not kill the mites themselves, so its effect is temporary. It can be sprayed on carpets or upholstered furniture to break down allergen from mites or cat dander. When the allergen is inactivated, it no longer causes allergy symptoms. Tannic acid works fast and is easy to use, but its effects do not last long because mites remain and allergen continues to build up. This requires frequent application of the product. Also, tannic acid may stain some carpets and upholstery so it should be tested in a non-critical area prior to widespread application.

Benzyl benzoate actually kills mites and helps remove them and their waste products from carpet. It comes as a moist powder that needs to be brushed into carpets, allowed to dry for 8 to 12 hours, and vacuumed up. Unlike tannic acid, benzyl benzoate's effect may be long lasting. After one or two initial applications, you might be able keep mites and allergy symptoms under control by using it only once or twice a year.

- **Pet Allergy**

Pets provide companionship, security and a sense of comfort. Children often learn responsibility and lessons about life and death from pets.

However, people with allergies should be cautious in deciding what type of pet they can safely bring into their home. Pet exposure may cause sneezing and wheezing. An estimated 10 percent of the population may be allergic to animals. A higher rate of 20 percent to 30 percent of individuals with asthma have pet allergies.

Pets can cause problems to allergic patients in several ways. Their dander, or skin flakes, as well as their saliva and urine, can cause an allergic reaction. The animal hair is not considered to be a very significant allergen. However, the hair or fur can collect pollen, dust, mold and other allergens.

What Are the Most Common Pets?

The most common household pets are dogs, cats, birds, hamsters, rabbits, mice, gerbils, rats and guinea pigs. Larger animals such as horses, goats, cows, chickens, ducks and geese, even though kept outdoors, can also cause problems as pets.

The number of pets in the United States is estimated at more than 100 million. This large number also increases the likelihood of accidental exposure to animals by the allergic patient when visiting homes, farms, etc.

Both feathers and the droppings from birds, another common pet, can increase the allergen exposure. The allergic patient should not use feather pillows or down comforters. If a feather pillow is used, it should be encased in plastic. An encasing with a zipper is recommended, so none of the feathers can escape.

Bird droppings can be a source of bacteria, dust, fungi and mold. This also applies to the droppings of other caged pets, such as gerbils, hamsters and mice.

What Do Allergists Recommend?

The best types of pets for an allergic patient are pets that don't have hair or fur, shed dander, or produce excrement that creates allergic problems. Tropical fish are ideal, but very large aquariums could add to the humidity in a room, which could result in an increase of molds and house dust mites.

A frequent misconception is that short-haired animals cause fewer problems. It is the dander (skin scales) that causes the most significant allergic reactions-not the length or amount of hair on the pet. As stated previously, allergens are also found in the pet's saliva and urine. In addition, dogs have been reported to cause acute symptoms of allergic conjunctivitis, or inflammation of the eye, and hay fever after running through fields and then coming back into contact with their owners.

Those pets that are known to cause significant allergic reactions should be removed from the home of the allergic patient to avoid possible progression of symptoms. A "trial" removal of a pet for a few days or even weeks may be of little value since an average of 20 weeks is required for allergen levels to reach levels found in homes without pets.

Can Pet Allergies Be Managed?

If the family is unwilling to remove the pet, it should at least be kept out of the patient's bedroom and, if possible, outdoors. Allergic individuals should not pet, hug or kiss their pets because of the allergens on the animal's fur or saliva.

Indoor pets should be restricted to as few rooms in the home as possible. Isolating the pet to one room, however, will not limit the allergens to that room. Air currents from forced-air heating and air-conditioning will spread the allergens throughout the house. Homes with forced-air heating and/or air conditioning may be fitted with a central air cleaner. This may remove significant amounts of pet allergens from the home. The air cleaner should be used at least four hours per day.

The use of heating and air-conditioning filters and HEPA (High Efficiency Particulate Arresting) filters as well as vacuuming carpets, cleaning walls and washing the pet with water are all ways of reducing exposure to the pet allergen. Vacuum cleaners with HEPA filters are now available. However, in a patient with severe symptoms resulting from animal dander exposure, a HEPA filter is not an effective solution.

Litter boxes should be placed in an area unconnected to the air supply for the rest of the home, and should be avoided by the allergic patient.

Some allergic patients may have severe reactions, such as wheezing and shortness of breath, after exposure to certain pets. Also, a chronic, slowly progressive feeling of shortness of breath, loss of energy and feeling of fatigue can result from long-term exposure to birds and their droppings. This type of disease is known as hypersensitivity pneumonitis and can result in severe disability. In the event of these severe cases, removal of the offending animal is mandatory.

How Are Pet Allergies Diagnosed?

The avid pet owner may claim that exposure to his or her pet does not cause their allergy symptoms. This, however, should be viewed skeptically, since pet ownership is an emotionally charged subject. Also, many allergic pet owners are rarely away from their pets, so an accurate reporting of pet-related symptoms may not be possible.

Skin tests or special allergy blood tests are helpful for diagnosing allergy to animals, but are not always accurate. To gain confirmation about a pet's significance as an allergen, the pet should be removed from the home for several weeks and a thorough cleaning done to remove the hair and dander. It should be understood that it can take weeks of meticulous cleaning to remove all the animal hair and dander before a change in the allergic patient is noted.

Are Allergy Shots Effective for Pet Allergies?

Allergy shots (immunotherapy) may be indicated for cat or dog allergies, particularly when the animal cannot be avoided-as might be the case when the patient is a small animal veterinarian. They are typically given for at least three years. They decrease symptoms of asthma and allergy. Usually after about six months of weekly injections allergy symptoms improve and less medication is required.

Allergy shots are most effective and safe when administered under the supervision of an allergist-immunologist. The response is highly individual and depends on environmental avoidance as well as the initial sensitivity of the individual.

What Can I Do When Visiting People With Pets if I Am Allergic?

The approach to visiting households with pets for an allergic individual is to take appropriate precautions including administration of medications prior to visitation. Your allergist-immunologist can provide information on medications for your animal allergy, such as antihistamines, nasal sprays, decongestants or appropriate asthma medications.

For patients who have severe symptoms on animal dander exposure, the pet should removed from the house at least day before the visit, and the host household should be cleansed of animal allergen to the extent practical.

- **About Food Allergies**

What Are Symptoms of Food Allergy?

Allergic reactions to foods typically begin within minutes to a few hours after eating the offending food. The frequency and severity of symptoms vary widely from one person to another. Mildly allergic persons may only suffer a runny nose with sneezing, while highly allergic persons may experience severe and life-threatening reactions, such as asthma or swelling of the tongue, lips or throat.

The most common symptoms of food allergy involve the skin and intestines. Skin rashes include hives and eczema. Intestinal symptoms typically include vomiting, nausea, stomach cramps, indigestion and diarrhea. Other symptoms can be asthma, with cough or wheezing; rhinitis, often including itchy, stuffy, runny nose and sneezing; and rarely, anaphylaxis, a severe allergic reaction that may be life threatening.

Because these symptoms can be caused by a number of different diseases other than food allergy, your allergist-immunologist may want to examine you to rule them out as the source of your problem.

What Causes My Symptoms?

A food allergy is the result of your body's immune system overreacting to food proteins called allergens. Normally, your immune system and defense mechanisms keep you healthy by fighting off infections and inactivating proteins such as food allergens, which could potentially cause allergic reactions. Therefore, the majority of people develop a tolerance to a wide variety of different foods in their diet.

In the individual with food allergy, the immune system produces increased amounts of immunoglobulin E antibody, or IgE. When these antibodies battle with food allergens, histamine and other chemicals are released as part of the body's immune reaction to these substances. These chemicals can cause blood vessels to widen, smooth muscles to contract, and affected skin areas to become red, itchy and swollen. These IgE antibodies can be found in different body tissues-skin, intestines and lungs-where specific allergy symptoms, such as hives, vomiting, diarrhea and wheezing are observed.

Not all adverse reactions to foods are due to allergy. Some reactions to cow's milk, for example, are related to a deficiency of an enzyme (lactase) that normally breaks down a sugar in milk (lactose). When individuals with lactase deficiency drink cow's milk or eat other dairy products, they may experience intestinal symptoms, including stomach cramping, gas and diarrhea. This is sometimes misinterpreted as a food allergy.

Why Me? Why Have I Developed Food Allergy?

Heredity seems to be the prime reason some people have allergies and others don't. If both your parents have allergies, you have approximately a 75 percent chance of being allergic. If one parent is allergic, or you have relatives on one side with allergies, you have a 30 percent to 40 percent chance of developing some form of allergy. If neither parent has apparent allergy, the chance is 10 percent to 15 percent.

Although food allergy occurs most often in infants and children, it can appear at any age and can be caused by foods that had been previously eaten without any problems. Finally, excessive exposure to a particular food may affect the overall rate of allergy to that food, as testified to by the high prevalence of fish allergy among Scandinavians and of rice allergy among the Japanese.

Which Foods Are Most Likely To Cause Allergy?

Eggs, cows milk, peanuts, soy, wheat, tree nuts, fish and shellfish are the most common foods causing allergic reactions, but almost any food has the potential to trigger an allergy. Foods most likely to cause anaphylaxis are peanuts, tree nuts and shellfish.

Keep in mind that, if you are allergic to a particular food, you might be allergic to related foods. For example, a person allergic to walnuts may also be allergic to pecans and persons allergic to shrimp may not tolerate crab and lobster. Likewise, a person allergic to peanuts may not tolerate one or two other members of the legume family, such as soy, peas or certain beans. Clinical research of individuals with food allergy, however, has demonstrated that the overwhelming majority of patients with food allergy are only allergic to one or two different foods. Complete restriction of all foods in one botanical family based on an allergy to one of its members is rarely necessary. Discuss these issues with your allergist.

How Do Allergists Determine Which Foods Make Me Sick?

Some people know exactly what food causes their allergic symptoms. They eat peanuts or a peanut-containing product and immediately break out with hives. Other individuals need their allergist's help in determining the "culprit", especially when the specific food cannot be identified or when the symptoms show up many hours after ingesting an offending food.

Your allergist-immunologist will typically begin by taking a comprehensive medical history. Specifically, you'll be asked about the symptoms you experience following the food ingestion, how long after the food ingestion they occurred, how much of the offending food was ingested, how often the reaction has occurred and what type of medical treatment, if any, was required. Moreover, you will be asked about your overall diet, your family's medical history and your home environment.

These questions are necessary because your allergist wants to eliminate the possibility that another problem or allergic condition may be causing or adding to your symptoms. For example, a patient's allergy to inhalant pollen such as ragweed may be related to allergic symptoms in the mouth and throat following the ingestion of certain melons, such as watermelon, cantaloupe or honeydew.

What Is Allergy Testing?

You may be asked to undergo some allergy testing. Your allergist-immunologist may employ skin testing, in which a diluted amount of the appropriate food extract is placed on the skin and the skin is then lightly punctured. This procedure is safe and generally not painful. Within 15 to 20 minutes, a positive reaction typically appears as a raised bump surrounded by redness, similar to a mosquito bite, and indicates the presence of allergic, or IgE, antibodies to the particular food. In some cases, an allergy (IgE) blood test can be used to provide similar information to that obtained by the skin test. The IgE blood test is generally more expensive than skin testing and the results are usually not available for one to two weeks.

If properly performed and interpreted, skin tests or IgE blood tests to foods are reliable and good screening tests for food allergy. However, it's entirely possible to test "allergic" to a food (by skin testing or IgE blood testing) and yet have no symptoms when that food is eaten. Thus, confirmation requires appropriately designed oral challenge testing with each suspected food.

How Do Special Diets Help Pinpoint the Problem?

With the information gained from your history, physical exam and testing, your allergist may further narrow down the suspected foods by placing you on a special diet. If your symptoms occur only occasionally, the culprit is likely a food that is eaten infrequently. Your allergist-immunologist may ask you to keep a daily food diary listing all food and medication ingested, along with your symptoms for the day. By reviewing and comparing "good days" with "bad days", you and your allergist may be able to determine which food is causing your reaction.

If only one or two foods seem to be causing allergic reactions, it may be necessary for the patient to go on a food elimination diet. The suspect food must be completely eliminated in any form for a short time-one to two weeks. If the allergic symptoms subside during abstinence and flare up when the food is ingested again, the likelihood of identifying the problem food can be increased.

If several foods appear to cause problems and/or the diagnosis of food allergy is equivocal, your allergist may want to confirm the role of each suspected food by oral food challenge testing. Not all positive skin tests and/or IgE blood tests equal a definite food allergy. With this in mind, food challenges are the best way to determine whether or not a food allergy really exists.

During an oral food challenge test the patient will eat or drink small portions of a suspected food in gradually increasing portions over a given period of time, usually under a physician's supervision, to see if an allergic reaction occurs.

Once My Allergy Is Identified, How Is It Treated?

Once the diagnosis of food allergy is confirmed, the most effective treatment is not eating the offending food in any form. Therefore, the patient must be vigilant in checking ingredient labels of food products and learning other names of identification of the responsible food or food additive to make sure it is not present. When you eat in a restaurant, you must be particularly vigilant and you should take emergency medicines with you if you have a history of severe reactions. Waiters (and sometimes the kitchen chef) are not always aware of the exact ingredients of each item on the restaurant's menu.

All patients with food allergies must make some changes in the foods they eat. Special food-allergy cookbooks, patient support groups and registered dietitians can provide valuable assistance regarding your diet. Your allergist can direct you to these resources.

What if I Accidentally Eat a Food I'm Allergic To?

Individuals with food allergy should have a clearly defined plan of action for handling situations in which they accidentally ingest a food allergen. Have a list of symptoms and your doctor's instructions for treatment posted in a prominent place in your kitchen. Oral antihistamines can be very useful in treating many of the early symptoms of a mild allergic reaction to a food.

Persons with histories of severe reactions need to be instructed in when and how to give themselves a shot of epinephrine (adrenaline) in the event of a severe allergic reaction. This medication is available in easy-to-use injectable devices and should be carried by persons with histories of severe allergic reactions. You should be taken to the hospital or call doctor and arrange for follow-up medical care for a severe reaction. Bracelets or necklaces may be worn to quickly alert medical personnel or other caretakers about food allergies.

Will I Ever Be Able To Eat These Foods Again?

In some cases, particularly in children, strict adherence to an elimination diet appears to promote the process of outgrowing a food allergy. For example, the vast majority of patients with documented allergic reactions to eggs, cows milk and soy eventually become tolerant to these foods. Allergies to peanuts, tree nuts, fish and shellfish, however, typically last a lifetime and are not outgrown. Overall, approximately one-third of children and adults will eventually be free of their allergic reactions to foods after rigorously following appropriate diets free of the offending food allergens.

After you have eliminated foods responsible for allergic reactions for a period of at least six months, your allergist may recommend that you undergo an oral food challenge under observation to reassess your symptoms. If you have no reaction and can ingest a normally prepared portion of the food, you will be able to safely reintroduce this food into your diet. If any symptoms of an allergic reaction do occur, the dietary restriction will need to be continued.

If you have had a severe immediate-type allergic reaction to a certain food, such as an anaphylactic reaction to peanuts, your allergist-immunologist may recommend that you never again eat this food and rarely would a food challenge be needed to confirm the history. Remember, in some very allergic persons a very small quantity of an allergenic food can produce a life-threatening reaction.

Patients who use caution and carefully follow an allergist's advice can bring food allergy under control. Please contact your allergist-immunologist with further questions and concerns about food allergy.

Latex Allergies

The incidence of serious allergic reactions to latex has increased in recent years. In rare cases, these reactions can be fatal. Health care workers and others who are frequently exposed to products containing latex should be aware of the potential for developing an allergic reaction. Individuals who exhibit symptoms of the allergy should be alerted to the need to limit future exposure to latex products.

What Is Natural Rubber Latex?

Natural rubber latex is a processed plant product derived almost exclusively from the tree Hevea brasiliensis found in Africa and Southeast Asia. Natural rubber latex should not be confused with butyl- or petroleum-based synthetic rubbers. Synthetic products, including latex house paints, have not been shown to pose any hazard to latex-sensitive individuals.

What Is Latex Allergy?

An allergy, or immediate hypersensitivity reaction, occurs when the body's immune system is sensitized to a foreign protein and reacts by forming a specific type of antibody, called an IgE antibody, specifically directed against this protein. This kind of antibody is responsible for a wide variety of allergic responses, which may range from hives to allergic rhinitis (hay fever), asthma, or rarely, life-threatening allergic attacks (anaphylaxis). These allergic reactions are provoked by exposure to common allergens including cat dander, ragweed pollen or antibiotics, such as penicillin. Latex allergic individuals make allergic antibodies directed against one or more proteins that are found in natural rubber latex.

What Triggers the Allergic Reaction to Latex?

When individuals allergic to latex come into direct contact with latex an allergic reaction may follow. Receiving medical or dental care from someone wearing a latex glove, blowing up a balloon, or breathing in glove donning powder are all common examples of circumstances where allergic reactions to latex have been triggered.

What Products Contain Natural Rubber Latex?

Latex is a common component of many medical supplies, including disposable gloves, airway and intravenous tubing, syringes, stethoscopes, catheters, dressings, and bandages. Many of these medical devices come into contact with mucous membranes, which enhances the absorption of latex proteins that can trigger an allergic reaction. Latex gloves also frequently are implicated in allergic reactions due to the repeated direct exposure of the wearer's hands to latex proteins or due to airborne latex proteins that are absorbed by powders used to lubricate some latex gloves.

While latex also is found in as many as 40,000 consumer products, including condoms, balloons, athletic shoe soles, tires, underwear leg- and waistbands, rubber toys, nipples, and pacifiers, these seem to only cause problems in the most sensitive patients.

What Are the Symptoms of Latex Allergy?

Allergy to latex proteins can cause symptoms similar to those seen in individuals who are allergic to bee venom or cat dander. Reactions on exposure to the allergen are generally acute and may mimic hay fever or asthma, with symptoms such as nasal congestion, hives or difficulty breathing. The most severe cases can result in anaphylaxis, a potentially fatal reaction that affects many parts of the body at once. Symptoms of anaphylaxis are usually immediate, progress rapidly and may include a dangerous drop in blood pressure, flushed skin, difficulty breathing, swelling of the throat, tongue and nose, and loss of consciousness. Emergency medical attention should be sought at the first sign of an anaphylactic reaction.

Skin problems resulting from the use of latex and non-latex gloves are frequently confused with latex allergy. Contact dermatitis is a frequent problem in glove wearers that can be caused by frequent hand-washing and drying with irritating soaps, skin abrasions from donning and removing gloves, and irritation of skin covered by an impermeable barrier. It can also be caused by contact allergy to one or several of the chemicals used in the production of rubber gloves. These are usually local skin problems but can involve larger areas. These local skin problems are not life-threatening, but may precede the development of latex allergy if latex exposure is continued.

How Do Symptoms Develop?

In most cases, latex allergy develops after repeated exposures to latex. It should be noted, however, that direct physical contact with latex-containing products is not needed to trigger the allergic reaction. Cases of anaphylaxis have resulted from inhaling latex proteins, which can be absorbed by the powder that is used to lubricate some latex gloves. When the gloves are snapped on and off, the proteins become airborne and can pose a risk to some individuals with latex hypersensitivity.

How Common Is Latex Allergy?

It is difficult to say how widespread the problem of latex allergy may be. More than 1,700 cases of latex allergic or anaphylactic reactions, including 17 deaths, have been reported to the U.S. Food and Drug Administration (FDA) since 1988. It is assumed that many other cases go unreported.

Known risk groups include:

- Health care workers and others who wear latex gloves.
- Individuals who have a history or who will be undergoing multiple surgical procedures, such as children with spina bifida.
- Individuals with a history of progressive allergic reactions to foods known to cross-react with natural rubber latex.

Other risk factors are less defined but appear to include a history of:

- Allergic rhinitis (hay fever) or any other allergy.
- Hand dermatitis, particularly if severe or if changing in severity in those who wears latex gloves.

Outside of these recognized risk groups, latex allergy is very uncommon, with estimates of less than 1 percent prevalence in the general population.

Why Is Latex Allergy More Prevalent Now?

The introduction of Universal Precautions in health care settings to prevent the spread of AIDS and hepatitis B resulted in a dramatic increase in glove usage. Latex gloves are the largest source of direct contact with latex products and the major source of latex aeroallergen in areas where powdered latex gloves are in use.

Who Is Most at Risk of Developing a Life-Threatening Anaphylactic Reaction to Latex?

The risk of anaphylaxis appears to be greatest in individuals with prior allergic reactions to latex-containing objects or prior, unexplained reactions or anaphylaxis during a medical or surgical procedure. Health care providers with a history of severe or worsening latex-glove-induced eczema, hives or work-related rhinitis or asthma-like symptoms should be especially cautious.

What Foods Are Known to Cross-React With Latex?

Some foods to which latex allergic patients frequently demonstrate sensitivity include avocado, banana, chestnut, kiwi, raw potato, tomato, stone fruits (such as peach, plum and cherry) hazelnut, melons, celery, carrot, apple, pear, papaya and almonds. Reactions are less common but have been reported to peanut, peppers, citrus fruits, coconut, pineapple, mango, fig, passion fruit, condurango bark and ugli fruit.

Reactions to many foods have been reported in latex allergic patients. In many cases, researchers have confirmed the presence of cross-reacting proteins with proteins found in latex. It is now thought that many of these allergenic proteins are plant defense proteins found widely in the botanical realm.

While food allergy is common in latex allergic individuals, neither the presence nor the distinct food allergies can be predicted for any patient. More severe latex reactions do appear to necessarily increase the risk of food reactions. Initial manifestations of food allergy can be severe and even anaphylactic. Latex allergic patients should have personal epinephrine syringes available at all times for this reason alone.

Patients with a history of food allergies to foods known to cross-react with latex rubber, particularly if expanding to new foods and progressive in severity, should be considered at risk for latex allergy as well.

How Can Latex Allergy Be Prevented?

All products and medical devices that come in contact with individuals at risk should be reviewed for possible latex content.

Respiratory exposure to latex proteins can take place in the absence of skin contact, since latex glove donning powders bind latex proteins in the gloves and carry them into the air. In recognition of this fact and that powdered latex gloves are the major source of latex aeroallergen, the American College of Allergy, Asthma and Immunology has issued a joint statement with the American Academy of Allergy, Asthma and Immunology calling for usage of only non-powdered low-allergen gloves. Synthetic and vinyl gloves may be acceptable alternatives.

How Can Health Care Workers Protect Themselves From Developing Latex Hypersensitivity?

Health care workers with a history of latex sensitivity who must wear gloves should stop wearing latex gloves, and their co-workers should not use powdered gloves. Care should be exercised in the choice of substitutes, since all synthetic or non-latex products are not equally impermeable to blood-borne pathogens.

Health care workers with a history of glove-associated skin irritations, or contact dermatitis, should use alternative gloves (which may include latex gloves) and topical treatments to relieve their symptoms. Petroleum-based products have been shown to compromise the barrier function of latex gloves, and care should be taken in the choice of treatments used to relieve contact dermatitis.

How is a Suspected Latex Allergy Confirmed?

An allergy skin test may be done to test for latex allergy, but there are currently no reagents commercially available for the test in the country. Recent research has demonstrated that latex skin testing with the material that is currently commercially available in Canada and Europe has better diagnostic sensitivity than the current available FDA approved blood tests. Because of the potential for a life-threatening anaphylactic reaction to the test itself, skin prick tests for latex allergy should be performed only under the close supervision of an allergy specialist. An allergist-immunologist also can order an IgE allergy blood test to confirm the presence of IgE anti-latex antibodies. Skin patch tests are used to evaluate the cause of skin irritations, or contact dermatitis, caused by chemicals inherent in rubber gloves.

How Are Latex Allergies Treated?

The best treatment for latex allergy is avoidance. Allergy specialists can provide latex allergic patients with information which will help them identify situations that place them at risk; strategies for avoiding an allergic reaction; and information about sources of natural rubber latex exposure and ways to avoid skin and mucosal contact.

Patients with latex allergy are at risk of asthma on exposure to latex-containing aerosols and should try to avoid areas where powdered latex gloves or their products are used.

Personal measures including warning bracelets and adrenaline syringes, like those commonly used for bee sting allergic patients, should be worn or carried at all times. Unexpected exposures to latex during dental, medical or surgical procedures may be prevented by warning health care providers of latex allergy prior to any scheduled visit and at the time of emergency visits.

Allergic reactions to a wide variety of fresh fruits, vegetables, legumes and nuts may complicate the course of latex allergy. Most commonly, banana, avocado, kiwi, hazelnut, raw potato, tomato, papaya, citrus, celery or stone fruits are involved.

Chapter 2

Antibiotics

Antibiotics—the wonder drug of the 20th century. These powerful drugs attack the bacterial infection in your system and within days the person afflicted feels remarkably better. Unfortunately these drugs require a dose of responsibility, and we have been taking them for granted for far too long. Nowadays it's all too common for a concerned parent to bring a child with a cold into the doctors' office and demand that they be put on antibiotics, and doctors are too often allowing themselves to be pressured into prescribing them. Each year about 50 million of the 150 million antibiotics prescribed to patients are unneeded for the illness to be cured. This needs to stop. Antibiotics are becoming obsolete because the bacteria they are fighting are becoming immune to them. The following will explain the current situation as well as provide tips and information about keeping your family safe from these "super bugs".

First off, it is important to note that ***Antibiotics only attack and affect illnesses caused by Bacteria.*** They are totally useless against viruses, and when used to fight a virus often only provide a way for the bacteria in the body to learn to resist the drugs and grow stronger. Some illnesses that you should take antibodies for are:

- Streptococcal sore throat
- Pneumonia
- TB (tuberculosis)
- Infections

- Lyme disease
- Legionnaires disease
- Meningitis (bacterial, not viral)
- Ear infections
- Sinus infections (some).

Illnesses that You Should Not Take Antibiotics for are:

- Bronchitis
- **Common colds** (in children 90% of colds and flus are viral)
- **Influenza** (the flu)
- Sore throats (with the exception of strep)
- Coughs.

However sometimes a viral illness will turn into a bacterial infection. when this happens consult your doctor. These are some signs to look for in children:

- Illness lasts longer than a week.
- High fever (which means your body is trying to fight back). If your child is younger than 6 months contact your doctor whether the fever is high or not.
- Sinus pain, ear or toothache develops.
- Cough of other symptom suddenly gets worse.

If you are prescribed antibiotics, it's very important that you do exactly as your doctor and pharmacist says. Take the pills when prescribed, and make sure you take the full dosage given to you. Stopping the medication early, even though you feel better is a bad idea as it is likely that only the weak bacteria would have been killed and the stronger bacteria has a chance to become immune to the antibiotics and return within a few weeks. Once this happens new drugs must be prescribed for you and your immune system will be weakened further. When your doctor tells you that you need antibiotics talk with them about it. See if you can take a shorter term prescription as opposed to a longer one, as shorter courses will give resistant bacteria less time to recover.

Be sure to ask about anything you're unsure of. It is also important never to take drugs prescribed for someone else.

Bacterial Resistance

So what is this resistance that keeps coming up? It's simple. It basically means that the antibiotics are no longer effective against these strains of the bacteria. This happens because in many cases not all the bacteria are killed after taking antibiotics-some of the strongest will survive. These few that survive become immune, or resistant, to the drugs. If the person gets ill again then they may need a different type of drug to cure the infection. The scary thing is that in 1994 some bacteria were found that could resist all available antibiotic drugs at that time-even the drugs used as a "last resort". Recently some illnesses that we thought we had defeated (TB) have come back, and this time they're able to resist our antibiotics. Because of this pharmacists and druggists have been working hard to come up with new drugs to protect us. Drug resistant strains can lead to prolonged hospital stays, complications and even death, and unfortunately drug resistant strains can spread fast. Currently about 30% of Strep throat infections are immune to penicillin, and the back up antibiotic, which forces doctors to use the "last resort" drugs, until recently the use of these drugs was rare.

If people start using antibiotics only when they really need them we'll see a drop in the resistant strains of bacteria and hopefully we will once again have a steady upper hand on the infections. As a parent you'll be able to better protect your family by keeping they're use of antibiotics to a minimum. Only give them antibiotics for bacterial infections, and if you can avoid using antibacterial creams, ointments and bandages on cuts and wounds. Sterilizing the wound will not help, and may in fact do more damage. Instead wash the wound with a water and salt solution. Also avoid things like harsh alcohols, peroxides, and detergents, as they are damaging to healthy cells. Once you've washed the wound with water or solution apply a regular bandage and it should be fine. If you start to see the early signs of an infection (swelling, redness, tenderness) then call up your doctor and they may advise you to apply an antibacterial ointment.

Another thing to be careful about is whom the antibiotics are being administered for. Elderly people may be affected in a negative fashion by the powerful drugs, as the side effects may keep them bed ridden or in pain. People who are very vulnerable to antibiotic resistant bacteria should be extra careful about the drugs they take to sure the infection. If the person in question is any of the following be extra careful and ask lots of questions when consulting a doctor.

- Premature infants and very young children
- Elderly
- Burn victims
- Bone marrow transplants
- People with weakened immune systems, such as AIDs, Leukemia, Cancer etc patients.

Medicine Safety

Understanding how your medicines work, and being alert to the following things can save your life, and help avoid medicinal mishaps. Medicine safety is no joke, read below for tips to keep you safe and informed.

When You are Still in the Doctor's Office

Questions to Ask Your Doctor and Other Tips...

- Ask your doctor for the medicine that offers the best balance of price and results or outcomes. This tells your doctor in a clear way that treatment goals need to be set, evaluated, communicated and achieved.

- If you're older (over 60) or have kidney disease be certain to ask if the new medications being prescribed will be removed by the kidneys. If this will happen your doctor will most likely want to adjust the dosage.
- Be sure to discuss with your doctor how often you'll need to take the medication. Be honest, if you don't think you'll remember three times a day perhaps there's another medicine for the same problem you'll only need to take once a day. You should "always" take your medicine as directed on the bottle.
- Ask for the name of the disease the medicine treats to be put on the label. This way if you're taking several medicines you won't risk getting them confused. It will also give the pharmacist an extra check when it comes to filling prescriptions and making sure they're giving you the correct drugs.
- You may wish to ask about side effects, if a certain drug will make you dizzy or tired and you need to take it in the mornings before work, you way want to try a different drug that will allow you to function properly. Some drugs have side effects that are worse than the thing they've been prescribed to cure, so knowing this may make you decide to use a different drug.
- It's also important to find out how soon you can expect to see results and what you should do if the medication doesn't seem to be working.
- While talking with your doctor, show him that you're really interested in your health, and making sure you understand what he or she is telling you. take notes, repeat directions and other information, and ask questions- even if you think they may seem foolish or trivial. Feel free to also inquire as to whether they have any printed information on your medicines on hand. It shows your doctor

you care and keeps you safe and informed. To make sure you don't forget something you may want to bring a list of questions with you before you visit the doctors office.

When You Go to the Pharmacy

- When your pharmacist hands you your prescription bag it's often stapled shut-open it up before you walk away. Inside it is your prescription and a brief patient info sheet. Your pharmacist can give you lots of information, and answer your questions about your medications. So if you have any questions about the medication, interactions, or other directions your doctor might have failed to mention, take this opportunity to ask them.
- Read the label when you look at your prescription. It seems simple, but many people don't do it. Reading the label will give you very valuable information—such as taking the medicine with food, and not taking it along with other medications. Ask if you should avoid certain foods, beverages, other medicines, or activities while you are taking the drug. Question anything you don't understand or that doesn't seem right. Be especially alert to unexpected changes, such as receiving a prescription refill that seems to have a different strength or appearance from your original prescription. If you have questions don't hesitate—Ask.
- Use the same pharmacy for all your medicines. Again this seems simple, but again it's something overlooked by many people. Using different pharmacies means that when having prescriptions filled for new drugs a single pharmacy might not have a list off all the medications you're currently taking. This makes it easy for mistakes to happen. You could be prescribed a medicine by one pharmacy that will interact with one you're already taking that comes from a different

pharmacy. Medicine reactions can be very dangerous, so use one pharmacy for all your medicine needs to keep yourself safe. It also gives you an opportunity to develop an good relationship with your pharmacist, they'll be familiar with your medicines which will further decrease the risk of error.

- Another way to avoid interactions is by having your medications mapped. This shows all the drugs you're taking, prescription, non-prescription and herbal, lists side effects, interaction notices, and maps out a logical daily routine for taking your medicine. All of this is on a single sheet of paper as opposed to the multiple pieces of paper that you get for individual prescriptions that you need to organize yourself. This is a fast and simple way to keep you safe and give your doctor and pharmacist and extra final check.
- If a medicine you're on is life sustaining, or you're deathly allergic to a certain type of medicine, you may want to invest in a medicine alert bracelet, tag, or card. These can be worn or kept in a wallet and if anything happens to you they'll let the medical response teams know what they need to do to help you.

When You Get Home

- Organize your medicines, if you've had them mapped then you've got a handy daily schedule telling you when you need to take your medicine. makes several copies of this in case one gets lost. If you keep a profile of the drugs you take be sure to keep it updated. Make a list of everything you're taking—prescription, non-prescription, herbal, medicinal foods, etc. and share it with your doctor and pharmacist this will help prevent drug interactions.
- Learn the names, doses, and strength, of the drugs you take.

- Take your medications exactly as your doctor and the label on the bottle prescribe. Doing this ensures that the medicine will work the way it's supposed to, and keeps you safe from bad interactions and other complications. Don't take to little, as it lessens the effect of the medicine, and don't take too much as it could be toxic. Occasionally missing a pill is also big deal/some medicines really do need to be taken every day, talk to your doctor to find out about how your medicines will react if missed. Also make sure that you finish a prescription you've been given unless instructed otherwise. If you're unsure if you were supposed to finish it or not call your doctor.
- If you realize you have more questions once you get home, don't hesitate to call your doctor or pharmacist. It is also important to call them before adding any other drugs (even non-prescription and herbal) to your daily drug regiment. If you're doctor or pharmacist won't make time to answer your questions you may want to consider finding some new health care providers who will make time for your questions—which are important.

Reactions

- If you think you may have had a reaction, no matter how minor—a headache which wasn't in the listed side effects, a sudden appearance of a rash, etc. call your doctor immediately to set up an appointment. If the reaction seems moderate to severe call your doctor or have a friend drive you to the nearest ER. Even if it turns out to be a false alarm, always be aware of things like that. Also, when you go to the doctor don't just tell them about the new medicine you've been taking, give them a list of everything so that they can check for drug interactions. If you've had a reaction your medications need to be changed, so don't hesitate. Minor reactions will get steadily worse and lead to bigger problems.

- If you are older and on medications, be careful. Some medications can make the elderly and those with a weak immune system miserable. The side effects of many drugs will leave these people bedridden, sick, and generally unhappy. the elderly especially are at risk because as you age your body adapts and reacts differently to medications. So if 6 years ago you took a medicine that worked for you very well, and you start taking it again, now as a senior citizen, you may see and feel considerably different. In situations like this you may not think to ask your doctor many questions about the drug because you've taken it before. But it's important to understand that while the drug hasn't changed your body has, and the two will interact differently and the medicine needs to be reevaluated to make sure it is the correct medication for your current state and situation.

Travelling Safely with Medications

- **Many medications can cause "photo-sensitivity," or increased sensitivity to sunlight.** Even if you don't usually **sunburn**, taking medications that cause this reaction could greatly increase your chances of getting a bad burn. Your pharmacist can advise you about whether your medication can cause photosensitivity and recommend the right SPF (skin protection factor) for your skin type.
- **If you are flying, keep your medications in your carry-on luggage so that you have access to them during your flight and will not lose them in the event that your luggage gets lost**. Plus, keeping your medications with you helps prevent exposure to extreme temperatures in the baggage

compartment, which can alter the drug's effectiveness. Keep in mind that airport security requires that your medications be transported in their original, labeled containers.

- **If your medication requires you to use a syringe/insulin, for instance/you may need to carry your prescription with you to ensure that you can pass through airport security.** The American Diabetes Association recommends that people with diabetes be prepared to provide airport security personnel with copies of prescriptions for diabetes medications and supplies as well as complete contact information for the doctor who prescribes the insulin.
- **Make sure that you carry your doctor's and your pharmacy's phone numbers with you when you are away from home.** In case you lose your medications, you may need a new prescription. You should also keep on hand a list of all your prescriptions.
- **If you are traveling through several time zones, consult with your doctor or pharmacist to work out a specific plan for adjusting the timing and dosage of your medications.** This will prevent you from taking too much or too little.
- **If you are visiting a foreign country, beware of buying "over-the-counter" medications.** Many medicines that are available by prescription in the United States are available "over the counter" in other countries. Some of these medications could have different ingredients, and may not undergo comparable quality control. Buying these medications could put you at risk for allergic reactions, drug interactions, or other problems.
- **If you are visiting a hot, humid climate, be sure to keep your medications in a cool, dry place out of direct sunlight.** Never store medications in the glove

compartment of your car. Also, because of the heat and humidity that build up in a bathroom, it is the worst place to store medication whether you are at home or on the road.

- Take along more medication than the number of days you've planned to be away. This will allow you to be prepared for unexpected delays.

Chapter 3

Back Pain

Back pain can occur due to various factors such as muscle strain, sprain or slipped disc. Being overweight can make back pain worse. One of the most common causes of back pain is doing work that you are not used to, such as carrying heavy objects or engaging in strenuous physical work.

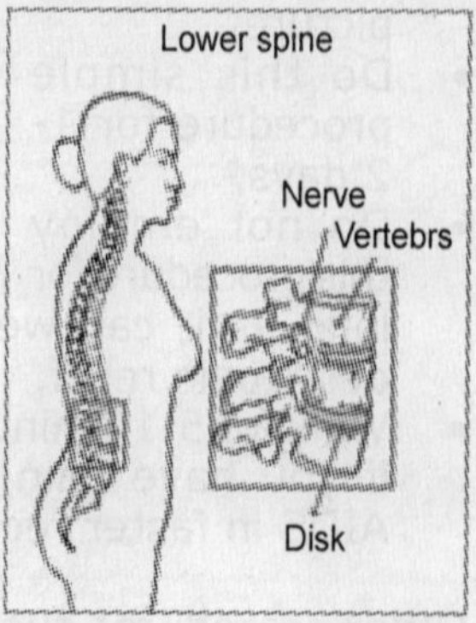

What is a slipped disc?

The bones that make up your spine contain disc-like structures between them. When a disc gets swollen and presses against the nerves, the condition is called slipped disc. It can be extremely painful and can affect the quality of your life.

The condition is usually caused while trying to lift heavy objects. Sometimes you may not be aware of the cause of your slipped disc. The good news is that slipped disc and other forms of back pain can be relieved by doing some simple exercises and/or medications. Getting your muscles in better shape and improving your posture when you are sitting, standing and sleeping can also help in preventing back ache.

Back pain relief

If you have hurt your back or are suffering

from a backache, *follow these steps to get some quick relief:*

- Lie on your back on the floor with pillows under your knees as shown in the picture.
- You may also keep your feet on a chair with your hips and knees bent as depicted in the picture.

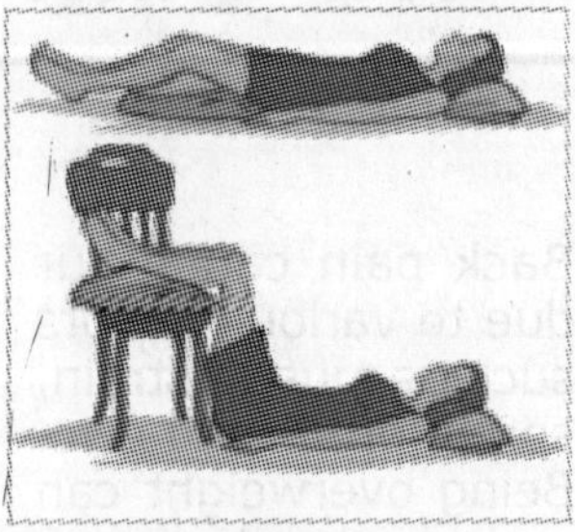

- Do this simple procedure for 1-2 days.
- Do not employ this procedure for long as it can weaken your muscles and delay pain relief.
- Walk for 5-10 minutes once in a while, even if you have pain, as physical movement AIDS in faster recovery.

Other procedures such as using heating pads, ice packs and body massages can also provide relief. But it is best to consult your doctor before using any of these procedures.

Seeking medical help

If you experience one or more of the following symptoms, get in touch with your doctor immediately:

- Your back pain spreads down up to your knees.
- You feel numb in your groin, rectal area, legs and foot.
- You have fever, weakness and sweating.
- The pain is so unbearable that you are not able to move.
- The pain does not go away even after 2 or 3 weeks.

Preventing back pain

The following tips will help you guard yourself from hurting your back:

- When you lift heavy objects, keep your

knees bent and squat while lifting the object. Do not bend to lift it.

- While carrying the object hold it close to your chest, keep your spine erect and straight.
- When you are lifting the object, do not twist your body.
- When you move heavy objects, push it instead of pulling it.
- Do not remain seated for long hours. Get up once in a while and stretch your body.
- Do not wear high heeled footwear.
- Exercise regularly. Lack of exercise can cause backache.

While standing

When you stand for long hours, shift your body weight from one foot to the other. You can also keep one foot in an elevated position by placing it on a stone, stool or raised platform. Stand straight and maintain a good posture.

While sitting

Use chairs with straight backs which provide adequate support to your lower back. When you want to turn, do so by moving your entire body. Do not twist your body at the waist. This can cause back strain. While driving, sit straight with your seat forward within easy reach of the controls.

While sleeping

Sleep on your side with your knees bent. Put a pillow under your head to support your neck. If you sleep on your back, put pillows under your knees and a small pillow under your lower back.

Finally

Certain exercises can help you strengthen your back. However, consult your doctor before doing these exercises; your doctor knows what is best for you.

Chapter 4

Bites

Bites of all kinds are serious, as bacteria and diseases are released directly into the body, and can spread quickly. Below is an outline of different kinds of bites and how to handle them.

Human bites: These should usually be treated as minor puncture wounds, and the area should be washed thoroughly with soap and water and then bandaged. Human bites can kill.

Marine creature bites: For bites and stings from creatures like jellyfish or Portuguese-men-of-war you need to be careful. Common jellyfish stings are usually not a big problem unless you are stung many times or are either very young or very old.

You handle jellyfish stings much the same way as a Portuguese-man-of-war (p-m-o-w) sting, even though p-m-o-w stings are more serious and can sometimes be fatal if you are stung too many times and do not receive the proper attention. Cover the jellyfish, or broken off tentacles with sand and very gently remove them and brush them off with a glove or piece of clothing. Do not touch them with your bare hands. P-m-o-w tentacles are paper thin, and even if they have broken off they will cling to you and continue to sting, hence the reason their stings are considered more harmful. It is possible to become ill from their sting, so if you've been stung by one make sure to seek medical attention quickly. If you are not hypersensitive to stings such as these, then you may treat these wounds as follows:

- Thoroughly wash the area and apply rubbing alcohol (or salt water) several times, while being careful not to touch the area with your bare hands.
- Coat the area in a thick layer of baking soda and water paste, which may be removed (scraped off) about 30 minutes later.
- Once you have removed the layer, you should reapply the rubbing alcohol or vinegar. Salt water will also work if you have neither at hand.

If a stingray has stung you, then seek medical help immediately. Wash the wound in fresh or salt water thoroughly and keep the wound submerged in hot water while you get help.

If a larger animal such as a shark, or other toothed creature has bitten you, refer to the animal bites section below:

Animal Bites: These can be superficial, but they can also be very serious.Most bite and scratches from household pets are superficial and can be treated with a simple washing of the wound, dab of antibacterial ointment and an adhesive bandage. But sometimes, Fido and Fluffy get a bit too frisky and really take a good bite out of you. When this happens, and when you are bitten by an animal that is not a pet of yours, you need to follow a different procedure.

- Wash the wound well with soap and water unless there is heavy bleeding. Then consult your doctor to determine if stitches are needed. If the wound appears serious do not attempt to clean it yourself.
- If the wound is large or deep you should see your doctor as soon as possible, as the wounds must be cleaned and bandaged properly to prevent the spread of bacteria and lower the risk of infection. If the wound is large and deep, stitches will be needed. In some cases, a tetanus shot and antibiotics will be necessary.

- If swelling, bruising, extreme pain, increasing redness (sometime seen as streaks), tenderness, warmth or drainage around the bite area occurs then consult your doctor immediately.
- Also any flu-like symptoms, such as fever, exhaustion, and swollen glands that occur soon after the bite or scratch should be reported to your doctor as soon as they appear. This is crucial as it could be signs of infection or a disease.
- If someone else's pet bit you, you must notify the owner and determine when the animals last rabies shot was. Vicious animals that were allowed to roam free should be reported to the local health departments.

Insect Bites and Stings

Signs and symptoms of an insect bite result from the injection of venom or other substances into your skin. The venom triggers an allergic (immune) reaction. The severity of your reaction depends on your sensitivity to the insect venom or substance.

Most reactions are mild, causing little more than an annoying itching or stinging sensation and mild swelling that disappear within a day or so. A delayed reaction may cause fever, painful joints, hives and swollen glands. You might experience both the immediate and the delayed reactions from the same bite or sting. Only a small percentage of people develop severe reactions (anaphylaxis) to insect venom. Signs and symptoms of a severe reaction include facial swelling, difficulty breathing, and shock.

Bites from bees, wasps, hornets, yellow jackets and fire ants are typically the most troublesome. Bites from mosquitoes, ticks, biting flies and some spiders also can cause reactions, but these are generally milder.

For Mild Reactions

- Move to a safe area to avoid more stings.
- Try to remove the stinger either with a tweezers or by scraping or brushing it off with a straight-edged object, such as a credit card. Swab the site with disinfectant.
- To reduce pain and swelling, apply ice or a cold pack.
- Apply 0.5 percent or 1 percent hydrocortisone cream, calamine lotion or a baking soda paste to the bite or sting several times a day until your symptoms subside.
- Take an antihistamine containing diphenhydramine (Benadryl, Tylenol Severe Allergy) or chlorpheniramine maleate (Chlor-Trimeton, Teldrin).

For Severe Reactions

Severe reactions may progress rapidly. Call doctor for emergency medical assistance if you experience any of the following signs or symptoms:

- Difficulty breathing
- Swelling of your lips or throat
- Faintness
- Confusion
- Rapid heartbeat
- Hives
- Nausea, cramps and vomiting.

Chapter 5

Blisters

A blister is a minor injury that unless it becomes infected, is found in unusual place, or reoccurs frequently can be treated at home without the assistance of a doctor. Blisters are formed by repeated the rubbing and friction in a particular area, which then fills up with fluid. Because they are so often exposed to friction the hands and feet are the most common place for blisters. Blisters will also form more easily on skin that is warm and moist, as opposed to dry or soaked, which again makes hands and feet an ideal place for blisters.

Types of blisters

There are two main kinds of blisters, friction and burn, and both are treated the same way. Leave the blister alone for a period of about 24 hours (you may cover it gently with an adhesive bandage to keep it from getting broken). If after this time the fluid has not been re-absorbed, and you can see no apparent change in larger blisters then you may begin the following treatment.

Over small intact blisters you should place a blister bandage and leave them alone, as they should heal quickly and you should not break them.

Larger intact (or ones with only a small tear) blisters are to be treated in the following way:

- Sterilize a needle or straight pin by heating it until it turns red in a flame, placing it in boiling water or soak it in rubbing alcohol.
- Clean the blister with rubbing alcohol or antibiotic soap and water.

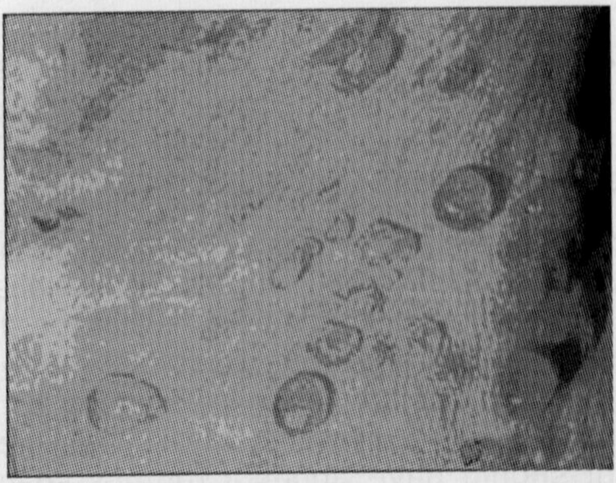

- After the needle has cooled, carefully pierce the blister on two opposite sides and press down gently on the blister with a sterile gauze pad to drain the fluid.
- Do not remove the loose skin!
- Cover the area with an antibiotic ointment. Keep in mind that you may want to avoid products containing Neomycin, which is known to cause allergic reactions.
- Then cover the blister with a blister bandage and change the dressing daily, or whenever it becomes wet, loose, or dirty.

Damaged Blisters

If the blister is has a large tear in it:

- Then take sterilized, fine scissors and carefully, remove the loose skin after the fluid has been drained.
- The area should then be thoroughly cleaned with antibacterial soap and water.
- Put on antibacterial ointment and cover with a blister bandage.

Infected Blisters

If you see any of the following signs your blister may have become infected and you should go to a doctor to receive the proper treatment.

- Pus draining from the blister.
- Very red or warm skin around the blister.
- Red streaks leading away from the blister.

Preventing Blisters

Blisters can be easily prevented, if the right steps are taken (no pun intended). For blisters on your feet, you should be sure that the shoes you buy are comfortable. The best time to buy shoes is in the afternoon or evening as feet tend to swell during the day. Shoes that fit right should have about a thumbs space in between your longest toe and the end of the shoe. If your shoes are too narrow they can cause blisters on your big and little toes, if the toe box is too shallow they can cause blisters on the tops of your toes, and if the shoe is too loose they can create blisters on the tops of your toes.

When buying shoes for a sport, make sure to wear the socks or padding you would normally wear around your feet to make sure that the shoe will fit comfortably. Jog or walk around the store before buying them and then wear them around the house for several hours to make sure they don't "rub" anywhere and cause uncomfortable friction.

Socks also help decrease friction in shoes, and socks made of synthetic materials remove moisture from the feet better than wool or cotton socks. This moisture removal also decreases the likelihood of getting a blister. If you know you feet will be sweating a lot, you can carry extra socks with you to change when the first pair starts to become uncomfortable.

Another step that can be taken to prevent blisters is to apply a thin layer of petroleum jelly to your feet. This will help decrease friction. This can also be used on your hands. Things like wearing gloves when doing activities such as construction, landscaping, moving, and other activities where your hands are exposed to friction will also help cut down on the likelihood of getting blisters.

Chapter 6

Breast Cancer

Breast cancer often presents itself as a hard, painless lump in one breast. Although breast cancer is rare under the age of thirty and very uncommon before the age of forty, the disease must at least be considered in any woman with a persistent breast lump.

If I detect a lump in my breast, could it be cancer

Breast lumps are among the most common complaints of women who visit gynaecologists. Whenever women feel their breasts, they are paranoid that they will discover a lump. It is probably because of this fear they feel they have detected a lump in their breasts every time they feel them. That can only mean one thing - the dreaded C word - cancer.

Three conditions must be distinguished in women with breast lumps: fibrocystic disease, fibroadenoma, and breast cancer.

a) **Fibrocystic Disease:**
Women with fibrocystic disease may feel many tiny cysts when they examine their breasts, and a consistency of lumpiness or doughiness.

b) **Fibroadenoma:**
Fibroadenomas are solitary, firm, mobile, benign tumors commonly found in young women in their twenties.

c) **Breast cancer:**
Breast cancer often presents itself as a hard, painless lump in one breast.

Is breast cancer common

Frequency of breast cancer in women is on the rise, partly due to the increased awareness of the disease and its diagnosis. It has also been seen that one in every eight women (or 12% of the women) will develop breast cancer.

What are the risk factors associated with breast cancer

- Highest risk factors
- History of breast cancer in a close relative (mother or sister)
- History of breast biopsy showing atypical cell growth
- Other Risk Factors
- First pregnancy after age 30, or no children
- History of breast cancer in a distant relative (maternal aunt or grandmother)
- Menstrual periods before age 12
- History of fibrocystic breast disease
- Obesity or a high-fat diet
- Menopause after age 50

Should I be worried about breast cancer

Breast cancer has accounted for over 17% of deaths in women. Depending on its severity, there are five stages of breast cancer.

In stage I, where the lump cannot be felt but can be diagnosed by a mammogram, the 5-year survival rate is 95%.

In stage II, where the malignant lump has not spread to the lymph nodes under the arm but has remained localized to one breast and is smaller than 2 cm, the 5-year survival rate is 85%.

In stage III, where the growth of the lumps is 2-5 cm and the lumps have not spread to the lymph nodes, the 5-year survival rate is 66%.

In stage IV, where the growth of the lumps is over 5 cm or the lumps have grown into the skin, the distant lymph nodes or into the chest wall, the 5-year survival rate is 41%.

In stage V, where the malignancy has spread to other parts of the body, the 5-year survival rate is 10% Persons at risk for breast cancer.

Is breast cancer hereditary

Yes. Breast cancer is a hereditary disease. If your close female relatives (like your mother or your sister) have breast cancer, then you face a greater risk of contracting the disease. However, given that you know you are in a high-risk category, it is possible for you to take extra precautions. You should be more vigilant about factors that are in your control - such as your childbearing age and your diet. You should also be more watchful about lumps in your breasts - both through regular self-examinations as well as through routine mammograms.

Is breast cancer age-related

Yes. The average age of women contracting this disease is 54. Women are also generally in the post-menopausal stage. It is very rare for breast cancer to affect women before the age of 35. Over 85% of tumors (benign or malignant) tend to develop in women above the age of 40. On the other hand, 30% of all breast cancers occur in women under the age of 50. It has been seen that close to 80% of the women who have breast cancer have no family history of this disease.

How is breast cancer screened

Early diagnosis is the key to treating breast cancer. Screening techniques are the closest you can come to prevention. This would involve monthly breast self-examination, periodic examination by your doctor, and selective use of mammography.

What is a biopsy

Although a doctor may suspect that a patient has breast cancer after examining her or after a mammography, the only way he can make a positive diagnosis is through a biopsy. This procedure involves removing a small sample of breast tissue and examining it under a microscope.

How can breast cancer be treated

There are several ways of treating breast cancer. The most common methods of treating breast cancer are surgery and chemotherapy. While carrying out a surgery, the aim of the surgeon is to remove as much of the infected tissue as is possible, without affecting the functioning of the neighboring muscles and tissues. This procedure is known as mastectomy. A simple mastectomy involves the entire removal of the infected breast.

Until recently, chemotherapy was only used for those in the advanced stages of the disease. Studies are now being conducted to determine the effectiveness of chemotherapy in the early stages of the disease also.

What is mammography and how is it performed

Mammography is a method of studying the breast with the help of X-rays. It is similar to taking X-rays of the chest or other areas. The difference is that a special, dedicated machine is required. Note that not all places that perform X-rays, can perform mammograms. During a mammogram, the breast is placed in a special holder, compressed and then X-rayed. Although there is mild discomfort, it is momentary.

Why should mammography be done

The only way to reliably detect breast cancer before it is palpable is by mammography. If this disease is detected early, it is less likely for the cancer to have spread. Local resection may be enough for treatment and the whole breast may not need to be removed. This also improves survival and prognosis.

When should mammography be done

All women over the age of 40 should have annual mammograms, irrespective of whether they have a breast problem. More importantly, mammography should be performed regularly on an annual basis. Mammography is also performed when there are symptoms related to the breast such as lumps, nipple discharge, pain, etc. Apart from this, if you have a first-degree relative (mother or sister) who has breast cancer, your risk of getting breast cancer is considerably higher. In this situation, an annual mammogram is mandatory.

Is any preparation required before taking a mammogram

No preparation is required, but it is advisable to wear loose clothing and not to apply anything to the breasts.

Treatment of Breast Cancer:

Surgery and Chemotherapy

What is a mastectomy

A mastectomy is a breast removal operation. Over the years, there have been many points of view propounded regarding the extent of surgery required.

The classical procedure was known as a radical mastectomy in which the entire affected breast, the chest muscles underneath, and the lymph nodes under the arm are removed. Most surgeons now agree that this is necessary only in rare cases. The standard operation for most breast cancers is now the modified radical mastectomy or the total mastectomy. In this procedure, the chest wall muscles are not removed. The simple mastectomy involves the complete removal of the breast, but not the lymph nodes under the arms or the chest wall muscles.

What is lumpectomy

Lumpectomy, otherwise known as a segmental mastectomy, involves the local removal of the tumor. In this procedure, only a portion of the breast is removed, including the cancer and a surrounding margin of breast tissue.

Lumpectomy accompanied by removal of the underarm lymph nodes coupled with subsequent radiation therapy is the popular alternative to a modified radical mastectomy. Radiation therapy is used after surgery to eliminate any cancer cells that may remain.

When should you undergo surgery

Surgery can be performed immediately after a positive biopsy so that the patient can avoid having to undergo a second round of anaesthesia and another surgery. Nowadays, the trend is to have two separate surgeries so that the women have time to evaluate their treatment options and seek a second opinion if they so desire.

What is adjuvant therapy (chemotherapy)

This treatment involves the use of chemotherapy (anti-cancer drugs) and hormone therapy. The role of adjuvant therapy is the subject of much debate. This treatment is usually prescribed at more advanced stages of the disease. In the future, the use of early chemotherapy and hormone therapy may be an important factor in reducing the death rate from this disease.

Chapter 7

Breathing Problems

Asthma

Asthma is a disease of the respiratory system. Your respiratory system is made up of your nose and mouth, your windpipe *(also called your trachea, pronounced tray-key-uh)*, your lungs, and a bunch of air tubes *(or airways)* that connect your nose and mouth with your lungs. When most of us breathe, the muscles that are wrapped around the air tubes *(airways)* are very loose and relaxed, and the lining inside the airways is very thin. This lets the airways open up very wide so that it is easy to get air in and out of the small air sacs that make up your lungs. These small sacs are called *alveoli (pronounced al-vee-oh-lye)*. When air moves in and out of your lungs, we call it ***breathing***.

An asthma attack is when something (such as dust, pollen, cigarette smoke) triggers a

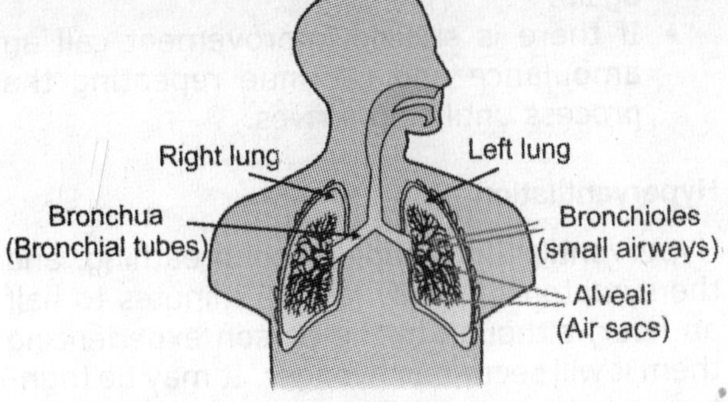

switch in the person that causes their air passages to constrict, tighten, and spasm causing the person to cough, wheeze and have difficulty breathing. They can also be caused by anxiety and tension. Most people who suffer attacks on a rather regular basis will carry their medication with them.

If someone you are with is having an attack:

- Help them assume an upright position, it will be for them to breathe than if they were lying down. You may want to encourage the person to sit with their legs crossed and their elbows on their knees as this is a relaxing position and may ease breathing.
- Talk to the person calmly and try to help them to relax.
- Make sure they are in an area where there is a good supply of clean air (as opposed to a dusty room).
- As soon as the person is sitting down, have them take their medication. If they cannot then you will have to assist them. Shake the puffer and give them one puff of reliever (with or without a spacer), they should then hold that breath for 4 seconds then breathe in and out normally 4 times. Repeat this step four times.
- Wait 4 or so minutes. If there is no improvement repeat the previous step again.
- If there is still no improvement call an ambulance and continue repeating the process until help arrives.

Hyperventilation

Hyperventilation is rapid short breathing, and the symptoms usually last 15 minutes to half an hour, although to the person experiencing them it will seem much longer. It may be frightening but hyperventilation is usually harmless and can be triggered by things such as:

- Anxiety (most commonly)
- Extensive physical injuries
- Severe stomach pains
- Heart or lung disease.

If you are Hyperventilating:

- Loosely cover your nose and mouth with a small paper bag.
- Slowly breathe into the bag and re-breathe the air in the bag about 10 times.
- Put the bag down and breathe normally for a few minutes before picking up the bag and repeating the previous step again.
- Repeat these steps until the symptoms lessen or go away.
- Try to focus on your breathing and remain clam. Try to take one breath every 5 seconds.

If Someone You Are With is Hyperventilating

- Stay calm and speak to the person clearly and slowly, if possible make eye contact.
- Don't crowd the person, give them space and make calming gestures and try to avoid making a scene. If they are not already sitting, have the person sit down.
- Encourage them to breathe normally, and walk them through the breathing cycle "breathe...slowly...hold...release...slowly ...rest...breathe..." and do the cycle with them. You'll want to pause for 1-2 seconds while holding the breath, and before inhaling again.
- If they are doing it right, calmly encourage them to keep going while continuing to breathe evenly and slowly.

Panic Attacks

Panic attacks are brought on by social situation and activities that are perceived as a threat to the person experiencing them. They can happen to anyone, and are usually not a serious threat. They can however occur rapidly and repeatedly, and even after the attack the person may be highly anxious for many hours afterwards.

Symptoms (not all will be present at once)

- Shortness of breath with rapid breathing, or hyperventilation.
- Palpitations or accelerated heart rate (when you can 'feel your heart pounding').
- Trembling or shaking.
- Choking.
- Chills, or flushing.
- Sweating.
- Nausea.
- Numbness, or pins and needles in the arms and legs.
- Chest pain or discomfort in the chest region (if pains persist after attack see a doctor, it may be signs of a heart attack).
- Fear of dying.
- Fear of going crazy or doing something crazy.

  You treat a panic attack the same way you would treat someone who is hyperventilating.
- Stay calm and speak to the person clearly and slowly, if possible make eye contact.
- Don't crowd the person, give them space and make calming gestures and try to avoid making a scene. If they are not already sitting, have the person sit down.
- Encourage them to breathe normally, and walk them through the breathing cycle "breathe...slowly...hold...release...slowly... rest ...breathe..." and do the cycle with them. You'll want to pause for 1-2 seconds while holding the breath, and before inhaling again.
- If they are doing it right, calmly encourage them to keep going while continuing to breathe evenly and slowly.

Chapter 8

Broken Bones

A broken bone is never a laughing matter and if you, or someone you're with, breaks a bone it's important to know what to do. Although you should **always** get medical help rather than trying to fix the problem yourself, sometimes help isn't available and you've got no choice but to try to help the person yourself. First off there are several different kinds of breaks. And before you begin any treatment, it's important to know what type you're dealing with. If you think an infant has broken a bone contact doctor immediately.

Classification

- A **Greenstick fracture** is when the bone only cracks, and does not fully break. Because these do not break the skin, they should be treated as a Single Fracture. These fractures can be determined by using X-rays.
- A **Bending fracture** occurs in children only. In this case the bone bends but does not actually break.
- A **Single fracture** is when the bone breaks in one place, and does not pierce the skin.
- A **Compound fracture** is when the bone has broken into two pieces.
- A **Comminuted fracture** is when the bone is broken in more than two places or crushed.
- An **Open** or **Compound fracture** is when the bone has actually punctured the skin and is visible. These breaks are very severe and have a high risk on infection. DO NOT

try to set these breaks yourself, instead get professional medical help immediately.

Once you've determined what type of break you have, there are a few things you should know about breaks in general. While your bones are strong, they can only take so much pressure and bend so much at one time before they crack or break. Younger people tend not to break bones as easily because their bones are more pliable, but bones that break at the ends should be looked at carefully because growth plates can be damaged. Older people are the opposite, a simple fall may result in a broken bone, which will take much more time and energy to heal. When a bone breaks, most people feel a sharp pain similar to that of a bad headache. The smaller the fracture the less pain you're likely to feel, this can make it confusing if you are trying to determine whether the bone is broken. Whether you think it is or not, ask your doctor because no matter how small a break it seems, a break is always a big shock to your body. With bad breaks, some people pass out because the brain gets sent too many signals at once, others feel pain or other sensations in parts of your body that are nowhere near the fracture. Other signs of a break are dizziness, sweating, thirst, pale or ashen skin, chills, and numbness or bruising around the fracture site. It is also important to try and get treatment for breaks as soon as you can because breaks that are not properly cared for can limit movement ability and cause deformities once they have healed.

How Do I Treat These Injuries?

Now here's what to do if someone has broken a bone. First and foremost, Stay Calm! Your staying calm will help to keep the person suffering the break stay calm and comfortable. Next, call your doctor or get to an ER. If you are out of reach (say you're camping in some remote area) and cannot get to help, or are instructed by a trained professional, only then should you begin the following steps. It is very important to note the following:

- If you think the person may have injured their back, neck, or head *DO NOT move them unless it is Absolutely Necessary!*
- Try not to move the broken limb, as it could cause more damage and pain.

If you cannot reach help, or have been instructed to administer aid, here are the following steps for helping the person in need:

1. Make the person as comfortable as possible before immobilizing the injured area.
2. To keep the area from moving you will have to make a splint. This works with leg and arm breaks where the arm is not bent. This can be done using a variety of materials such as boards, rolled newspapers, sticks, an umbrella, rolled blankets etc. Place the item around the injury and gently secure it with rope, strips of cloth, a tie; whatever you have available.
3. If the above materials are unavailable, and the injury involves limbs, you may tape or tie the injured leg to the uninjured one, tape an injured arm to the chest, or to the side of the body (surround the limb with padding first) depending upon whether the elbow is bent.
4. After you have wrapped and splinted the limb, check for a pulse. If you cannot find one then it means the bonds are too tight and must be loosened. Because fractures cause swelling you should check this often to make sure the person remains comfortable. Other signs that the splint is too tight are a numbness, tingling, or bluish tint to the skin at the sight of the break.
5. If the person has broken their arm and the arm is bent at the elbow then take a cloth and fold it into a triangle. Then gently

slip the widest part under the arm and tie the two ends around the neck, forming a makeshift sling. You want the arm resting at a 90° angle.

6. To keep the swelling and pain down, apply an ice pack, ice wrapped in a cloth, or, if all else fails, a bag of frozen vegetables. Do not keep the ice on for much longer than 20 minutes as it can cause numbness and discomfort.
7. Unless the person is bleeding, aspirin, ibuprofen, or another pain reliever may be used to ease the pain.

Healing Process

Once you have received professional help for a broken bone, the healing process can begin. Some bones are placed in a sling, others in a cast and depending upon the severity of the break can be in a cast for a few weeks or several months. Sometimes with more severe fractures, where the bone is crushed or broken into several pieces a steel pin is used to help repair the bone and set it in place. When the cast comes off you may notice that the area underneath the cast looks pale, dry, and smaller (where the muscles are). Don't worry this is only temporary. It's good to remember that even though you are out of a cast or sling, your bone is still very weak and sensitive and it's a good idea to avoid sports and activities where you might re-injure yourself until your doctor tells you it's OK.

Safety Tip/Prevention

When you're able to get back into the sports arena, remember, to avoid breaking another bone always play it safe! Wear any protective gear available when participating in any activity that can cause serious injury. Helmets, pads, face guards, and most importantly Seat Belts! Many states these days make wearing your seat belt a law, but don't just do it because it's the law, do it because it could save your life! If you're driving a car and want to cut down on the risk of serious injury in case of an accident, make sure all your passengers are buckled up before you start the car. Remember, it's not just a safety tip... it's the law!

Chapter 9

Burns

What Are Burns?

Burns are injuries that damage and kill skin cells. These wounds often need special consideration and require a trip to the doctors. Burns can be caused from hot liquids and materials, common household chemicals, fire, radiation from the sun, and other sources. When someone has been burned there are three important factors that must be looked at, depth (first, second, or third degree), area (total body space covered), and location (where the burn is on the body).

Depth is a measure of how deep the damage to the skin goes. We will look deeper into the three degrees of damage in the section below. The total body area is also important, the skin is a barrier to protect the body, and when it's damaged, the victim is subject to fluid loss and infections. If more then 15% of the body surface is damaged the victim can go into **shock**, and may require hospitalization for IV fluid resuscitation and skin care. The most important factor is location. If a burn occurs on the neck or near the nose and mouth, the persons breathing passages may be affected. Burns often swell and this could become a life-threatening problem if the airways become constricted. Another facial burn that needs special attention are the eyes. These should be looked at as soon as possible and handled very seriously as burns to the eyes may lead to clouded or lost vision. Because burned tissues shrink, burns that extend circumferentially around body structures often require the surgical removal of the dead and damages tissue, this procedure is called an escharotomy. Burns are often difficult to heal and may leave scars.

Burn Prevention

Burns of all kinds can be prevented easily. Keep household chemicals out of reach of children. Make sure hazardous chemicals are well marked and caps are screwed on tight. Keep hot object safely out of reach and make sure to turn off heaters and stovetops when finished to prevent burns. Also keep socket caps over all unused electrical sockets to protect against electrical shock, and keep all electrical wires away from water.

Classification and Treatment

First Degree

Most first degree burns are superficial and can be cared for at home without the help of a medical professional. These burns are much like typical sunburns and are cared for in a similar way. You should immerse the burn in cool water (do not use ice!) and then blot it gently and apply burn cream and then cover with a dry, clean, non-stick pad.

These burns usually leave the skin red and mildly swollen. The skin sensations are intact and the burn is painful to the touch. Most average sunburns are characterized as first degree burns.

Second Degree

Second degree burns are more serious and should be seen by a medical professional. If the burn seems very severe report to an emergency room or call your doctor. Although second degree burns often look like first degree burns, in the sense that they are red, the damage goes deeper. With these burns, the pain is more intense and blistering may occur. The burns may also be wet, or weeping and may have a shiny surface. It is advised that these burns are not touched or covered.

Third Degree

These burns are the most serious. Third degree burns are very deep and the burn often appears white, deep red, or black because of skin death. These burns are often without sensation because nerve endings have been damaged. It is important that these burns are not touched, or covered unless absolutely necessary. Any contact with the burned skin can cause more damage and heighten the chance of infection.

- For both second and third degree burns.
- If face is affected sit the victim up and watch for breathing difficulties, until medical help is received.
- If arms and legs are affected, keep them elevated above heart level.

Burn Treatment

- Remove any constricting jewellery.
- Do NOT use oils or butter on a burn.
- Douse effected area with cool water (Except in the case of a bad third degree burn) ASAP!
- Do NOT use ice or ice cold water, this can cause additional damage.
- Cover the wound with a **Hydrocolloid**, these dressing are a natural way of letting your body heal itself and are gently on your skin. When hydrocolloid needs to be changed (when it becomes saturated) it will fall off. In the cases of bad burns, contact your doctor before administering any first aid.

If you have not received a tetanus booster within 5 years, get one to protect against tetanus infections.

Electrical Burns

If someone receives an electrical burn, they should seek professional attention immediately. These burns often result in serious muscle breakdowns, electrolyte abnormalities, and occasionally kidney failure. An important thing to note about these burns is that the damage is often internal and cannot be seen from the outside.

Electrical burns occur when there is contact with electricity, either alternating current (AC) or direct current (DC).

Caring for an Electrical Burn

- Call or send someone to call 911 for emergency medical assistance. Significant electrical injuries will need medical care.
- Unplug the appliance or device that has caused the injury or turn off the electrical current.
- If the child is in contact with the electrical current do not touch them until you turn off the source or the circuit breaker.
- Determine that the child is still breathing. If the child is not breathing, begin cardio-pulmonary resuscitation (CPR).
- Cover the burned area with a sterile gauze bandage or clean bed sheet.
- Maintain your child's normal body temperature, and take the child to an emergency center.
- Be aware that a child may experience "shock" (see below) after an electrical burn. If your child is showing signs of shock, send someone to call 911 immediately.
- Do not give your child anything to eat or drink.
- Place the child on his/her back, unless a neck or back injury is suspected.
- If the child has vomited or has a serious injury to the face or mouth area, you may lay the child on his/her side.

- Keep your child warm with blankets or extra clothing, but do not use a heat source to warm them.
- Elevate your child's feet and legs, using a prop or pillow.

Chemical Burns

These burns should be treated like thermal burns and doused with large amounts of water to flush out the effected area. Contaminated clothing should be removed. It is also very important that you DO NOT try to neutralize the chemical burn by adding another chemical, as this could result in a chemical reaction causing thermal burns or greater skin damage. Many chemicals can be treated to reduce skin damage, so when in doubt it's a good idea to call your local poison control center or make a trip to the local ER. When working with chemicals always wear the proper protective gear to avoid burns and other injuries.

Sun Burns

A sunburn is the result of your skin being exposed to too much of the suns ultraviolet radiation. This threat varies greatly with the seasons and with changing atmosphere conditions. The amount of sunlight you are exposed to also depends on the geographic features of altitude and latitude, as well as clothing, lifestyle and occupation. Indoors, sunburn-producing rays are filtered out by ordinary window glass. Outdoors however the suns rays are able to pass through light clouds, 25 cm of clear water, and fog.

The telltale signs of sunburns appear between 1-24 hours. If the burn is light, the skin will be red, swollen and will hurt when touched. If the burn is more serious it will be very painful to the touch and blisters may develop along with redness and swelling. If a large portion of the body is burned chills, fever, weakness and even shock may be experienced. Treat your burns with care. Aloe Vera is a healthy moisturizer and help soothe the pain and heal the skin. Other gentle moisturizers such as Noxzema may help cool and soothe the itching and pain. Anesthetics may be used to ease pain, unless blisters are present. If used around blisters they may make the problem worse! Also be careful as local anesthetic lotions may cause a sensitizing reaction. As the burn heals the burned skin peels off and new skin is revealed. This skin may be hypersensitive for the next few weeks and care should be taken.

Healing Tips

- Drink lots of liquids.
- Taking a hot shower after receiving a mild burn can bring about peeling sooner.
- Vitamins E and C can be ingested as part of a daily diet or spread as an ointment over the burn. This will help prevent severe damage from the burn and shorten its effects.
- Aloe Vera will also help sooth the pain of sunburns.
- Another simple and easy summer pain reliever for sunburns is watermelon rind. Cut away the pink fruit and place the greenish white rind over the burn, it has a cooling effect and will temporarily relieve the discomfort of the burn. Not to mention the yummy treat will be a great distraction from the pain!

Sunburn Prevention

The best way to deal with sunburns is to avoid them in the first place. Using sunscreen is a simple way to protect yourself that takes little time and will be invaluable towards keeping your skin looking healthy. For most people, SPF 15 is strong enough to protect them from burns, but if you burn easily (lighter skin) then remember that the higher the SPF the stronger the protection. For most sunscreens to work at their best, they should be applied at least 30 minutes before going out since they take about that much time to bind to your skin. This is especially important if you'll be in the water or participating in some high-energy activity where you will perspire. Many people think sunscreen is just a summer product, but in fact it is helpful all year round. During the summer, exposure to the midday sun should not exceed 30 minutes, even if you tan before you burn. In the winter the greatest danger comes on foggy days when the UVB levels are almost as high as on clear days, this danger is greater at higher altitudes. Use Scivolutions, Inc. **"ItSUNuff"** sun exposure monitor patch to tell when you have had enough sun and should get inside before you burn.

Chapter 10

Carbon Monoxide Poisoning

What is Carbon Monoxide?

Carbon Monoxide (CO) is a colorless, odorless gas that is very dangerous to living things. Inhaling these fumes disallows proper oxygen transport in the body and can do serious damage to the central nervous system. Inhalation of too much Carbon Monoxide can be fatal. People who already suffer from health problems (such as heart or lung diseases), the elderly, pregnant women, children and infants are especially vulnerable to serious injury from inhalation.

Where Does It Come From?

Carbon Monoxide is a gas that is created when something is burned such as:

- Wood
- Gasoline
- Coal
- Kerosene
- Natural gas
- Tobacco smoke
- Un-vented heaters
- Automobile exhaust
- Blocked chimney
- Malfunctioning cooking appliances
- Malfunctioning gas, oil, wood, or coal furnaces/fireplaces
- Malfunctioning gas dyer
- Malfunctioning water heater
- BBQ grills, heating units, or pool/spa heaters that lack proper ventilation.

Symptoms

CO poisoning mimics many other common illnesses, and often many people do not realize they're in trouble until there's a serious problem. Not all symptoms will be present and different people will experience them differently. The most common are:

- Drowsiness
- Weakness
- Dizziness
- Disorientation
- Blurred vision
- **Headaches**
- **Nausea and vomiting**
- **Seizures**
- Rapid heartbeat
- Cardiac arrest
- Respiratory failure
- Loss of hearing
- Loss of consciousness or coma.

Treatment

If you think you may have inhaled carbon monoxide fumes see a doctor ASAP to make sure that no damage has been done.

Prevention

- Have your fireplace or furnace cleaned and inspected each year before you start using them again.
- Use non-electric space heaters only in areas where there is good ventilation.
- Do not use non-electric portable heaters or lanterns while sleeping in enclosed spaces, such as tents, campers, other vehicles, and rooms with no ventilation.
- Do not leave a running car or other vehicle in an enclosed area whether you are working in there or not.
- Remember that at higher altitudes you are at a greater risk of being affected by these fumes sooner.

Chapter 11

Chickenpox

Chickenpox is a common disease caused by the varicella-zoster virus (VZV), which is part of the herpesvirus family. Although many people associate the word herpes with genital herpes, the herpesvirus family is made up of nearly 100 kinds of viruses, eight of which cause disease in humans. Examples of different herpesviruses are herpes simplex virus (which causes cold sores and genital herpes infections), Epstein-Barr virus (which causes infectious mononucleosis), and varicella-zoster virus (which causes chickenpox and shingles). Varicella-zoster virus spreads in the air through coughs or sneezes or through contact with fluid from inside the chickenpox blisters.

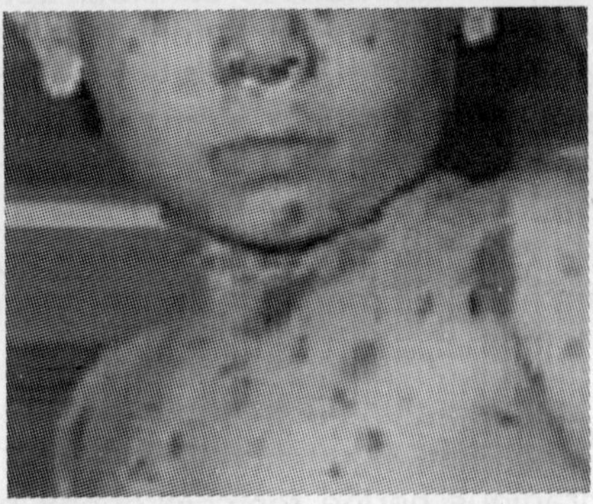

Chickenpox which occurs most often in the late winter and early spring, is very contagious- if exposed to an infected family member, about 80 to 90% of those in a household who haven't had chickenpox will get it. However, immunization of children with the chickenpox vaccine that's now available is expected to decrease cases of the disease dramatically over the next few years.

Although it's more common in kids under the age of 15, anyone can get chickenpox. A person usually has only one episode of chickenpox in his or her lifetime. But the virus that causes chickenpox can lie dormant within the body and can cause a different type of skin eruption later in life called shingles, also referred to as herpes-zoster

Chickenpox is an incredibly common viral illness that runs rampant with children, despite the fact that most children are now vaccinated as toddlers against the disease. The illness is best known by its notorious red and insanely itchy rashes that tend to spread all over the body. These red rashes will advance to fluid filled blisters, which will drain and scab over. Luckily, with the exception of those who are allergic to chickenpox, people only have to suffer through this disease once. Once you've caught it, your body develops lifetime immunity to the virus. If as an adult you've never had this virus you may want to consider getting a vaccination for it, as cases among older people can lead to complications. Getting a vaccine is an especially good idea if you're thinking about starting a family and have never had chicken pox. If you're older and you catch the disease you want to be very careful and act quickly. Adults are at risk of complications such as pneumonia, bacterial infections etc.

Contagiousness

The contagious period for chickenpox begins about 2 days before the rash appears and lasts until all the blisters are crusted over. A child with chickenpox should be kept out of school until all of the blisters have dried, which is usually about 1 week, but you don't have to wait until all the scabs fall off to let your child get back to a normal schedule.

Pregnant women, as well as people with diseases or problems with their immune system, should *not* be near a person with chickenpox. If a pregnant woman who hasn't had chickenpox in the past contracts it (especially before 20 weeks), the fetus is at risk for birth defects. If she develops chickenpox 5 days before to 2 days after delivery, the newborn is at risk for life-threatening varicella (the mother has transferred the virus to the baby, but she hasn't had time to produce and transfer antibodies, which fight off infection, to the baby before it's born).

If the mother had chickenpox in the past (before the pregnancy or any time more than a week before delivery), then the fetus receives antibodies through the placenta. That means the mom's immunity gets passed on to the baby through the placenta and breast milk, so it would be unlikely for the infant to get sick. But antibodies are not fail-safe; there is no 100% guarantee that a baby won't get the infection-it's just less likely. Or, the infant might have the disease, but it won't be as severe. It's also important for pregnant women to realize that *they're* at increased risk of chickenpox complications if they catch it for the first time while pregnant.

People who haven't had chickenpox can also catch it from someone with shingles, but they cannot catch shingles itself. Why can't a person catch shingles from someone else? It's because shingles can only develop from a reactivation of the varicella-zoster virus in a person who has previously had chickenpox.

Chicken Pox Spreads in the Following Ways

- Like a cold, it can be spread through sneezing, coughing etc.
- Contact with clothing or other linens the person has touched.
- Or by touching the person, or the blisters on the person who's suffering from the virus.

- The person will be most contagious the day before the rashes first appear and the following 7 days after they first appear. The incubation period of the disease is 7-21 days.

Treatment

- If your child has the chickenpox, keep them out of school! The virus is incredibly contagious, so be aware if your child has friends who have developed the pox, as it is likely your child will develop it soon as well. By being tuned in to this you can help prevent more children from catching the illness. Keep your child home until most of the scabs have formed and fallen off.
- You can ask your doctor to provide you with some antihistamines to help relieve the pain and swelling of the rashes.
- To cut down on the number of rashes, don't let your child itch them. Have them wear mittens or socks on their hands and keep their fingernails trimmed.
- Sometimes other things happen as a result of the chicken pox, like a bacterial skin infection, or pneumonia. If either of these arises your doctor will have to prescribe some **antibiotics** to deal with the problem.

Prevention

Since 1995, a *varicella vaccine* has been given to children older than 12 months, as well as adults. The vaccine is about 70 to 85% effective at preventing mild infection, and more than 95% effective in preventing moderate or severe disease. People who do develop chickenpox after vaccination have much milder symptoms with fewer skin blisters and a fast recovery.

The vaccine is recommended to be routinely given to children at 12 to 18 months of age. Older children, adolescents, and adults who haven't had chickenpox should also be immunized. Whereas children 12 months to 12 years receive a single vaccine dose, adolescents and adults require two vaccine doses a minimum of 4 weeks apart. Considering that the vaccine could prevent illness and even deaths, not enough children are being vaccinated, according to the Centers for Disease Control and Prevention (CDC). As is the case with all immunization schedules, there are important exceptions and special circumstances. Your child's doctor will have the most current information.

There's also a second type of prevention for certain people who are at risk for severe disease and who've already been exposed to the infection. A ready-made form of immune protection called varicella-zoster immune globulin (VZIG) is given to newborns whose mothers had chickenpox at the time of delivery; high-risk patients (such as those with leukemia or immune deficiencies); and kids receiving drugs that suppress the immune system.

Healthy children who have had chickenpox do not need the vaccine-they usually have lifelong protection against the illness. However, 10 to 20% of people who've had chickenpox develop shingles later in life.

Incubation

The incubation period for chickenpox is 10 to 21 days after exposure; most cases appear in 14 to 17 days. For example, if one child in a family breaks out with chickenpox picked up at school, siblings probably will show symptoms about 2 weeks later.

Duration

Chickenpox usually lasts 7 to 10 days in children, but typically lasts longer in adults.

Professional Treatment

A virus causes chickenpox, so your child's doctor won't prescribe antibiotics (which are for bacterial infections). However, your child may require antibiotics if the sores become infected by bacteria, a common complication.

An antiviral medicine known as acyclovir may be prescribed for anyone over the age of 12, people with weakened immune systems (from diseases or medications), and those with long-term lung or skin diseases. The drug, which can make the chickenpox less severe, must be given within the first 24 hours after the rash appears. Acyclovir is *not* prescribed for children younger than 12 because the drug can have side effects. Your child's doctor can tell you if the medication is right for your child.

Home Treatment

Most home treatment is aimed at relieving the annoying itch of chickenpox and the accompanying fever and discomfort. However, **NEVER use aspirin to reduce pain or fever in children with chickenpox or certain other viral illnesses.** Using aspirin in such cases has been associated with a serious disease, called *Reye syndrome,* which can lead to liver failure and even death.

Some measures you *can* take to help your child get through this itchy, uncomfortable time:

- Use wet compresses or give baths in cool or lukewarm water every 3 to 4 hours for the first few days. Oatmeal baths, available at the supermarket or pharmacy, can help to relieve itching. (Baths do *not* spread chickenpox).
- Pat (don't rub) the body dry.
- Put calamine lotion on itchy areas (but don't use it on the face, especially near the eyes).
- Give your child foods that are cold, soft, and bland because chickenpox in the mouth may make drinking or eating difficult. Try to avoid feeding your child any-

thing that's highly acidic or especially salty, like orange juice or pretzels.
- Ask your child's doctor or pharmacist about pain-relieving creams you can apply to sores in the genital area.
- Give your child acetaminophen (such as Tylenol) regularly to help relieve pain from mouth blisters.

And although it's tempting, children should be discouraged from scratching. Tell your child to come to you for help when faced with the urge to scratch. In addition, trim your child's fingernails and keep them clean to help lessen the effects of scratching, including broken blisters and infection.

When to Call Your Doctor

Most chickenpox infections require no special medical treatment. Call your child's doctor immediately if your child:
- Has fever that lasts for more than 4 days or rises above 102 degrees Fahrenheit (38.8 degrees Celsius).
- Has a severe cough or trouble breathing.
- Has an area of rash that leaks pus (thick, discolored fluid) or becomes red, warm, swollen, or sore.
- Has a severe headache.
- Is unusually drowsy or has trouble waking up.
- Has trouble looking at bright lights.
- Has difficulty walking.
- Seems confused.
- Seems very ill or is vomiting.
- Has a stiff neck.

Call your child's doctor if you're uncertain about whether your child's problem is chicken-pox, if you have a question, or if you're concerned about a possible complication. The doctor can guide you in watching for complications and in helping you choose medication to relieve your child's itching.

Chapter 12

Choking

Heimlich Maneuver

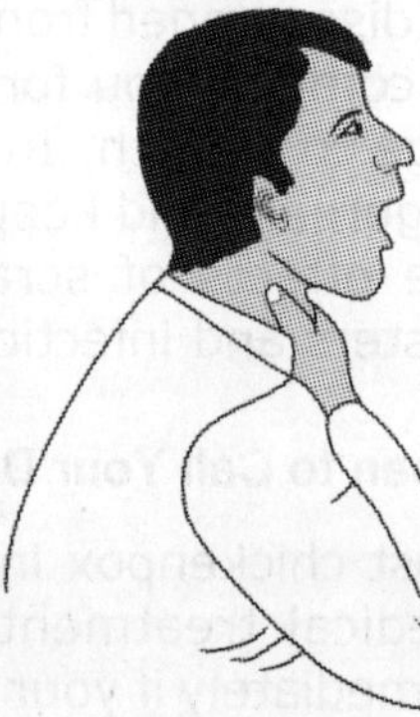

This maneuver is used to stop someone from choking on a foreign object blocking the airway by removing the object. This simple first aid procedure forces air out of the lungs in an attempt to force the obstruction out of the airways. This procedure should be used on all conscious choking adults and children from ages 1-18. If the child is under a year old, the method is not recommended and should not be used. The Heimlich maneuver is a series of under the diaphragm abdominal thrusts, which force air from the lungs to create and artificial cough. This "cough" is intended to remove the obstruction from the airway. Each thrust should be given in attempt to remove the obstruction.

Although the Heimlich maneuver is simple and effective, it can be painful for and even injurious to the victim. It's something to be reserved for genuine emergencies, and should be performed only when the situation meets the following guidelines:

- The person cannot **talk**, **cough,** or **breathe**. (If the person is coughing, they're not choking, so don't perform it).
- The person nods yes to the question, "**Are you choking?**"

- The person is **unconscious** and your attempts to breathe for them are blocked.

Method 1: Perform it on a Conscious Person

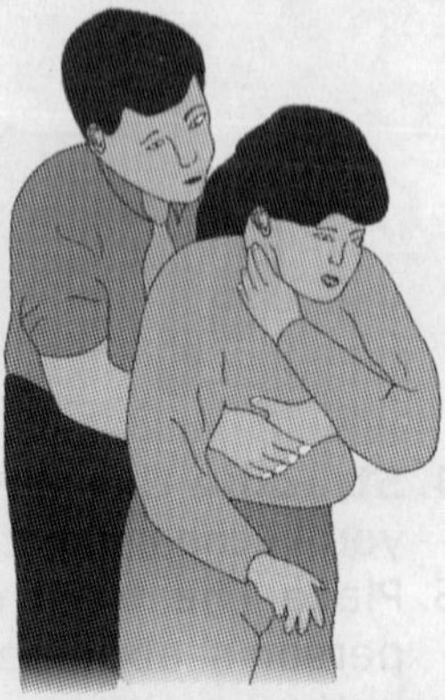

1. Stand close behind the victim with **your thigh between their legs**. Some experts recommend that you stand sideways behind the victim (with your hip at a 90 degree angle to the victim's back). This enables you to brace your hip against their lower back or buttocks.
2. **Make a fist** with one hand, and place it thumb-first against the person's abdomen, **an inch (about 3 cm)** above the belly button.
3. Cover that fist with your other hand. Keeping your elbows out, sharply and quickly pull your fist **inwards and upwards**.
4. Be sure to perform this motion with sufficient force to dislodge the object; it often must be repeated **up to six times**. If the object remains stuck, lie the person on their back, and continue as if the person were unconscious. If someone else is present, have them call your doctor. If you're alone, proceed directly to **Method 2.**

Method 2: Perform it On An Unconscious Person

1. Lower the person to the floor and **onto their back**. If another person is present, have them call your doctor.
2. **Open** their mouth and try to see the object.
3. **Sweep** your hooked finger across the back of their throat. Remove the object if you find it.

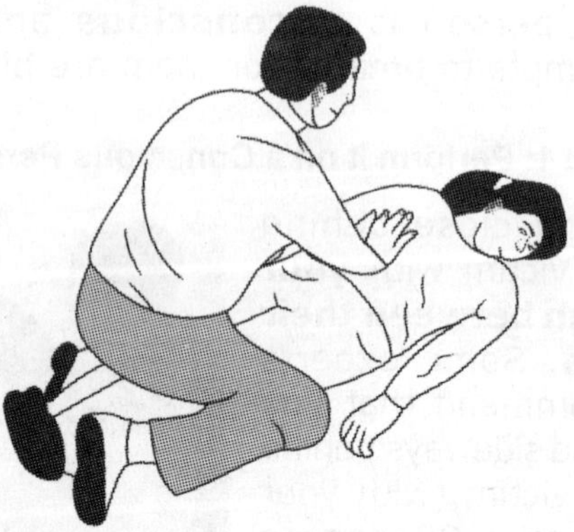

4. **Straddle** the person's thighs. This will put you in the correct position to do the thrust.
5. Place **the heel of your hand** over the person's abdomen just above their belly button, and cover that hand with your other one.
6. Keeping both arms straight, press **down, and forward** into the abdomen with a quick thrust.
   It may be necessary to repeat this up to four more times.
7. If the object hasn't popped out, again sweep your hooked finger across the back of their throat. Remove the object if you find it. **Call** your doctor**.**
8. **If the person vomits**, turn them on their side to avoid further blockage of the air pipe.

Method 3: Perform First Aid for A Choking Small Child or Infant

Small children and infants have much more fragile bodies than the rest of us. The two methods below are designed to minimize damage to very young bones and tissue. Go to **Step 2** if only if **Step 1** is ineffective.

1. **Find** a chair and sit on it.
2. Place the child/infant **face-down across your lap**, with their upper torso hanging over the side of your knee.

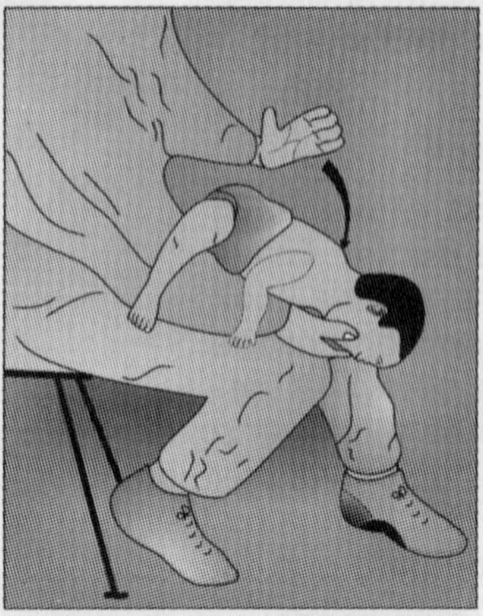

3. Using the heel of your hand, thump the child/ infant firmly but gently **four times** between the shoulder blades. Be especially careful with infants. Increase the amount of force only if a gentle thump doesn't dislodge the object.
4. If you haven't dislodged the object with several thumps, call your doctor. If the victim is an infant or very small child, go on to **Step 2**.

The "Upside Down by the Ankles" Method

1. Hold the victim **upside-down by the ankles**. You'll need to hold the both ankles in one hand, with your thumb around one leg, your three last fingers around the other leg, and your index finger in between their legs.
2. Thump the victim's back **between the shoulder blades** firmly but gently.

Caution: Don't search blindly in a small child or infant's mouth. You can accidentally push the object further down their throat. (Although you should remove the object if it's readily visible.) If the child vomits, turn their head to the side to keep them from choking further. If the child is unconscious, **call your doctor.**

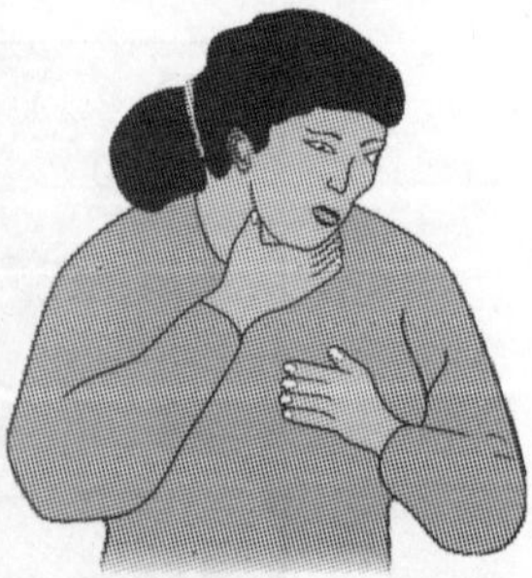

Method 4: Perform it on yourself

Your first move is to call your doctor. Leave the phone off the hook and perform one of the methods below. It requires some willpower to administer this painful technique on yourself, but your life may be at stake. You have a bit less than two minutes before you pass out.

Use your own hands

1. Make a fist with one hand, and place it **thumb-first** against your abdomen, just above the belly button.
2. Cover that fist with your other hand, and pull your fist **inwards and upwards** sharply, quickly and forcefully. Repeat several times if necessary.

Use A Sharp-edged Object

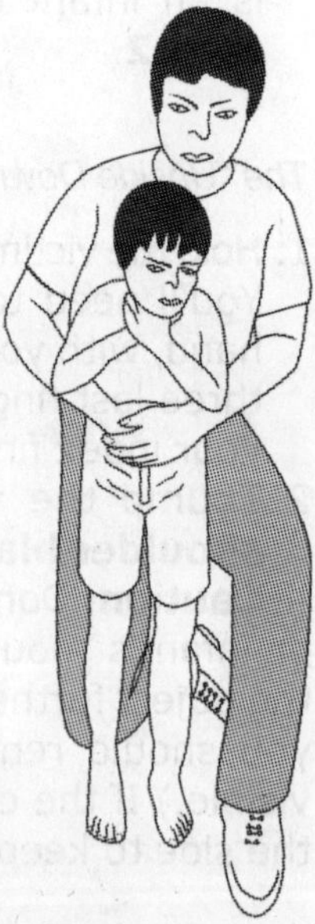

Use this method if **Step 1** doesn't dislodge the object.

1. Locate **a straight-backed chair** and place it firmly against a wall or angle it in a corner.
2. **If a chair isn't available**, use a sharp counter top, deck railing, staircase railing, or the sharp edge of a table, stove, or piano.
3. Run into the object. Attempt to meet it at the spot **just above your belly button**. Run at the object repeatedly and with as much force as you can muster until the object is dislodged.

The Heimlich maneuver is simple and effective on choking victims when used by itself. If you also know **CPR**, you'll have another powerful life-saving technique to use on an unconscious person. Your local hospital or city administration offices should be able to provide you with the location of CPR classes near you.

Chapter 13

Cold Injuries

Cold injuries, such as frostbite and chilblains are common during the winter months when people are out exposing themselves to the elements. Many people think that for a cold injury to occur the temperature has to be below freezing (0°C, 32°F) but in fact cold injuries can occur in temperatures above freezing if there's a wind chill or when a glove or sock gets wet. There are two types of cold injuries, the ones where body tissues freeze and the ones where they do not. The people most susceptible to cold injuries are the young and the elderly, although anyone who exposes him or herself to the cold is at risk.

Cold Injury Classification

No tissue freezing

Chilblains: These are the most common cold injuries. They tend to occur when there is exposure of skin to a dry cold. In this case, the affected area may itch and appear reddish blue and be swollen and painful. Over time blisters containing clear fluid may form and the area will be sensitive to cold in the future. Luckily there is often no permanent damage.

"Trench Foot": The name of this condition comes from the cold injury that often took hold on the soldiers living in the trenches during World War I. This condition also goes by the title of Immersion injury. These injuries occur when a part is the body is exposed to a cold

and wet environment. For example, if while playing out in the snow your socks get wet you are increasing your risk of developing trench foot is you fail to correct this problem. These are like chilblains, except they are often more serious. The blisters are deeper and resemble those of burns, and the area remains sensitive to the cold. Again there is usually no permanent damage.

Tissue freezing

Frostbite: This is probably the most serious cold injury. In this injury the tissues of the affected area actually freeze. Ice crystals form within the cells, causing the cells to rupture and die. Luckily this injury has several stage and can be caught early.

The first stage is called "frostnip" this occurs when only the surface skin is frozen. It starts like a chilblain, with itching and pain. The skin then progresses to loose it's blood supply, and eventually looses feeling and goes numb. Because only the top layers of skin are affected, there is usually no permanent damage aside from long-term sensitivity to cold, which may occur.

The second stage occurs if no action is taken in the situation described above. In this case the skin becomes hard and frozen , luckily deep tissues are spares and remain soft. Several days (usually 1-2) after the injury occurs, hard blisters will form. They often appear blackened and look worse than they are and heal within about 3-4 weeks. These injuries should usually be seen by a doctor and again the only permanent damage is heat and cold sensitivity.

If the injury progresses to the third (or fourth, depending on severity) stage of frost-bite then the deep tissues are affected. Here the muscles, tendons, blood vessels and nerves of the affected area are frozen. The area will feel hard and woody and you may not be able to move the part on it's own (for example, if your fingers are affected you will lose the use of them). This loss of use may be temporary or in serious cases permanent. The affected area looks either deep purple or red with blisters, which are usually filled with blood. Frostbite such as this usually results in the loss of fingers and toes. Often it may take several months to determine the extent of the damage, and surgery is usually delayed until they are certain that the tissues cannot be revived.

How Do I Treat These Injuries?

There are a few important things to remember when treating these injuries the first of which is vital. It is very important never to thaw an affected area if there is a risk that it may re freeze. If it is warmed then refrozen ice crystals will form and more damage will be done. If you are afraid the area will become re frozen then leave the affected area frozen. Another mistake would be to follow the old folk remedy of rubbing the affected area with dry snow. Any rubbing may aggravate the area and cause more damage. Warming the injury is the proper treatment but cold injuries should never be warmed over a fire or next to a heater. This could cause painful burns and dry out the injured tissues, causing again, more damage.

The proper way to treat these injuries is to put the affected area into a tub of hot water (104-108 degrees F and 40-42 degrees C). It is very important to take the temperature of the water with a thermometer or a hand that is not frozen. It is very important to avoid burning the injured area, and it may not always be obvious because these areas often lack feeling. When feeling is returned there may be quite a bit of pain in some cases. Aspirins, ibuprofen, and acetaminophen may be used for the pain. If you feel stronger pain control is needed contact your doctor.

Who is Most at Risk?

As mentioned above the young and elderly are at the greatest risk. The elderly have poor circulation and children have smaller limbs which freeze much faster. In both cases they may not be able to get help or recognize the problem before the injury is upon them. Other people at risk are those who consume alcohol during the cold winter months and those who are taking medications that depress the ability to feel naturally. These people may not recognize they are in trouble until it is too late. Alcohol causes warm blood to become cooled at the surface of the skin, which sets the person at a greater risk of getting a cold injury. And lastly those who have illnesses such as diabetes, poor circulation, hypothyroidism and arterio-sclerosis are at a greater risk as well.

How Do I Prevent A Cold Injury?

The best way to prevent these injuries is simple. Dress warmly and move indoors when your fingers, toes, or face begin to feel cold. Always keep your hands and feet dry and covered, and change wet gloves and socks as soon as possible. It's also good to keep your ears covered. Several drugs have also been tried to prevent frostbite by dilating the blood vessels and increasing circulation but the effectiveness of these is anecdotal, and it has not been proven to help. Medications to avoid are beta-blockers. These medications reduce circulation and increase the risk of cold injuries.

When is Medical Help Advised?

Chilblains can usually be treated at home, while a doctor should look at trench foot and frostbite cases. Those two injuries require long-term evaluations to watch for complications. Infection of a cold injury is often increasing redness and warmth. Also, if there is a lot of blistering and you are not up to date on your tetanus shot, you should get a booster. If you are unable to get medical care for your chilblain cold injury, try to keep the **blisters** closed, and clean. If they do open let them drain then cut off any dead tissues with a pair of sterile scissors. Once the blister is open, it is important to keep it clean and covered. A first aid cream such as bacitracin may be used.

The Common Cold

The common cold is a common annoyance to millions of people each year, particularly in the winter months. The cold, which can be caused by hundreds of different viruses, is an incredibly infectious respiratory infection that usually lasts about a week or so. Once you've become infected with the virus, it will take a couple days before symptoms start to appear. Once they do, be careful! the first three or four days of a cold are when you are contagious and most likely able to pass it on to other people. In most cases an over the counter medication is sufficient, but if you're afraid it may be a bacterial infection consult your doctor. The symptoms of the common cold are as follows:

Symptoms

- A 'sick' 'under the weather' feeling
- Sneezing
- Head and chest congestion
- Runny nose
- Post-nasal drip
- Sore throat
- Stiff joints and muscle aches
- **Headaches**
- Sleepy, weary, worn out
- Chills
- **Fever** (usually small)
- Watery eyes.

If any of these symptoms are present along with some the ones above you may have **Meningitis** get emergency medical help immediately.

- Seizures.
- Red blotches on skin, different from being flushed, look Somewhat like wounds. (Septicemia).
- Pale blotchy skin (in young children).

Also Seek Professional Advice in these Cases

- If an infant (under 3 months) is showing any of the symptoms.
- If your throat is very sore, you have a high temperature and symptoms seem to be getting worse.
- If you're having trouble breathing, or are wheezing.
- If your temperature is very high-this may be a sign of pneumonia, get help immediately.
- If you are pregnant or breastfeeding.
- If the cold lasts for longer than 2 weeks and symptoms seem like they're getting worse.

Treatment

Besides handy over the counter medications (Triaminic, vapor rubs etc.), and lozenges (cough drops) for a sore throat there are many other things you can do to fight off a cold.

Vapor: By inhaling some vapor, you'll loosen up some of the congestion, which will make it easier to breathe and will help to clear out your system. Heat up some water so that it's steaming, and keep it near you so you can inhale the fumes. This may make it easier to fall asleep at night. You can also sit over the fumes, and by placing a towel over your head and the bowl you create a tent where the fumes are trapped. If the fumes are hot enough you'll kill some of the germs off as well.

Foods: Fruits and vegetables are a must. Spicy foods may also help to clear out your system, as will garlic and onions. Avoid dairy products as they'll lead to the formation of more mucus, and try to leave large amounts of egg, starch, and sugar out of your diet for a while as well. If you're feeling nauseous avoid anything greasy. Try and eat nutritiously, it'll help you get better faster and make you healthier so that you have a better chance of fighting off future colds.

Drink: Water, water, everywhere-that's what you need to drink. Water helps you flush out your system, so it's absolutely vital to drink when you've got a cold. Juices, especially citrus drinks, are also good for you. Hot tea, will make you feel better as well-it's tasty and it has vapors which will help clear your nasal passages. Again avoid dairy. If you're nauseous a small amount of a slightly sweet soda-like ginger ale-will help settle your stomach.

Other: If you like natural remedies, try some Echinacea at the first sign of symptoms. This will stop the infection from reaching it's full potential and will therefore reduce the severity of the cold. Also avoid things like cigarettes during this time as they may aggravate your condition.

Prevention

It's difficult to avoid the common cold-particularly during the cold season-but you can do many things to lessen your chances of contracting it.

- Keep yourself healthy. Good diet, exercise, avoid smoking and drinking.
- Wash your hands often-germs can survive for a few hours without a host, so anything you touch that someone who is sick has touched has potential to get you sick.
- If you're already sick cover your mouth and nose when you sneeze and cough, and keep your own hands clean. This will help stop the spreading of germs.

Causes

Colds and flues are generally Kapha (phlegm) diseases. Exposure to cold air, seasonal changes are Kapha increasing factors. Exposure to hot and cold conditions alternatively in a short period is also responsible, as for example having cold water or drink immediately after coming in from the sun.

Remedies

- An anti-Kapha diet should be taken. It should be warm, light and simple. Dairy products according to Ayurveda are Kapha promoting and should be avoided.
- Lemon and ginger juice can be taken with warm water and honey three times a day.
- A good formula can be made with equal parts basil, sandalwood and peppermint, 2- 3 tsps. put them in a cup of water bring to boil and then have it upto three times a day.
- Sitopaladi powder is an extremely effective remedy for common colds and problems of sinus congestion. The dose is 1-5 gm with honey, three times a day.
- Sweating is very helpful. One simple method is to induce sweating is to drink a hot cup of tea, and lie down in the bed and take some blanket and let the body sweat for 15-20 minutes.

What Causes a Cold?

The common cold is caused by any of a number of viruses that can involve the upper respiratory tract. As your body reacts against the attacking virus, you get the symptoms of a cold—including nasal congestion, sneezing, and sniffles.

What Causes the Flu?
What's the Difference Between Respiratory Flu and Intestinal Flu?

Influenza, or "the flu", is caused by one of several strains of the influenza virus. These viruses usually cause symptoms in the head and chest—such as congestion, sore throat, or cough—but also can cause intestinal symptoms such as nausea and vomiting. The influenza virus also can have general symptoms such as fever, muscle aches, chills or sweats.

Are People with Strong Lungs—Runners or Dancers, for Instance—Less Susceptible to a Cold or the Flu?

Regular exercise, from aerobics to walking, boosts the immune system. People who exercise may still catch a virus that causes a cold or the flu, but they may have less severe symptoms and may recover more quickly than their friends who do not exercise.

Are People Who Have Asthma or Allergies at Greater Risk for Catching A Cold or Flu?

Yes. People who have asthma or allergies may already have inflamed and irritated lungs. Their bodies are already fighting one irritant or illness, so it is often more difficult for them to fight off a virus. Smokers are also more likely to have irritated lungs and are thus more likely to catch a cold or the flu.

Are You Contagious Before You Show Symptoms? If a Co-worker is Sniffing Over the Phone You Share, Is He or She Contagious Then?

The viruses that cause colds and the flu are spread by microscopic droplets from an infected person's respiratory system. It may be possible to catch the virus before symptoms show, via close contact such as kissing or sharing eating utensils. However, people generally need to have some symptoms, such as a runny nose or cough, in order to be contagious. When your co-worker shows symptoms, he or she may indeed be spreading contagious droplets to your shared phone, to the doorknob of your office, or to the buttons on the fax machine. Your best defense is to wash your hands frequently.

Chapter 14

Concussions

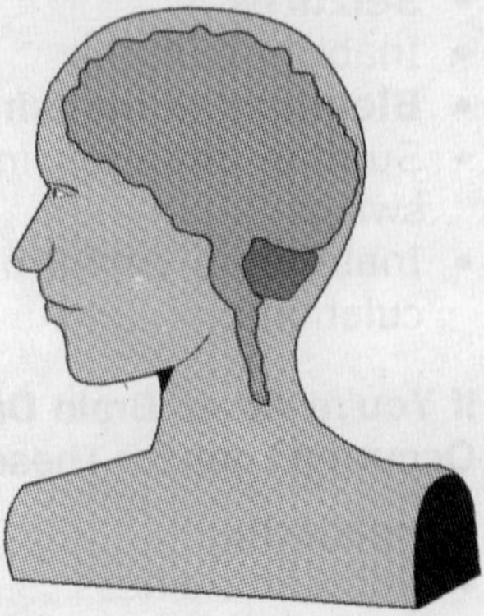

A concussion is by definition "any impact to the head". The impact to be worried about is anything that hits you in a moderate to quick motion. When this sort of impact happens the brain may collide and bounce off your skull. This causes swelling to occur and in severe cases, it causes a bruise to appear on the brain known as a contusion. Because brain tissues are so sensitive and delicate moving around in this fashion can cause them to tear, stretch, twist, and swell. When these things occur the "messaging' system of the brain is often disturbed and the person may have trouble with certain mental or physical activities. Whiplash, car accidents, blows to the head, falls, and (most common) sports injuries are all common causes for concussions. Sometimes when a person receives a concussion they will go unconscious, this is often a sign of brain damage and should be dealt with promptly.

Signs of a Concussion are as Follows:

- Blurred vision
- Slurred speech

- Delayed (or incoherent) verbal and motor responses
- Drowsiness
- Confusion
- Memory loss
- Persistent headaches
- Dilated pupils
- Uncoordinated movement
- Loss of balance
- **Seizures**
- Inability to focus
- **Bleeding or bruising** behind the ears
- Sudden changes in personality or mood swings
- Inability to perform simple tasks and calculations.

If You're Afraid Brain Damage May Have Occurred Look for These Signs:

- Headache
- Unconsciousness
- Pale skin
- Unequal size of pupils
- Difficulty speaking
- Clear or reddish fluid draining from ears, nose, or mouth
- Paralysis of an arm or leg opposite the side of the injury to the head
- Paralysis of the face on the same side as the head injury.

While Waiting for Medical Assistance to Arrive

It seems as though the person has suffered more than just a bump on the head, and you have called for medical assistance you may perform the following steps to help the person:

1. While waiting for medical assistance lay the victim lying down in the recovery position. (Head lowered and legs elevated, loosen any tight clothing, apply cool, damp cloths to face and neck (if available).

2. Make sure the victim is breathing properly.
3. Control any *bleeding.*
4. If the victim becomes unconscious for any amount of time, make sure to note this information and report it when medical help arrives.
5. Even if they complain of thirst do not give the victim anything to drink.

Prevention

Someone who has suffered several concussions could be at a higher risk of facing problems with vision, balance, memory, and concentration later in life. The damage from concussions is accumulative, which is why it's extra important to wear the proper head gear when participating in sports or activities where you might be in harms way. To avoid whiplash injuries always buckle up when you get into a car.

Chapter 15

Conjunctivitis (Eye Flu)

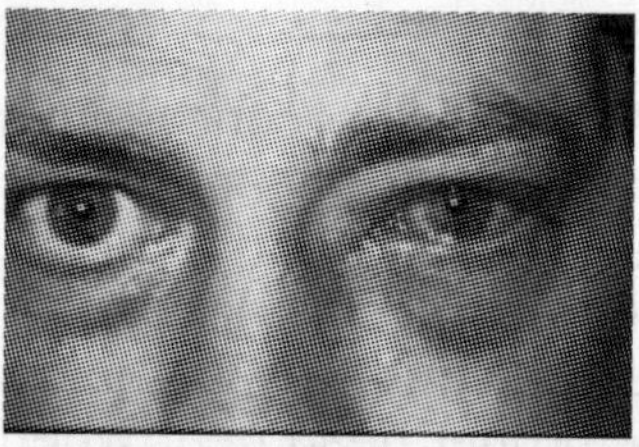

Conjunctivitis is the inflammation of the delicate membranes around the whites of the eye and is commonly caused by either a bacterial (pinkeye) or viral infection or as a result of allergies. In most cases this condition is not serious and can be treated at home. However, if the situation has not improved within 5 days you should call the doctor. Although not all the symptoms will appear together-some you'll find in relation to allergy, others in connection with bacterial infections-here are some signs to look for.

Symptoms

- Tears
- Swollen lymph nodes
- Burning, and very itchy eyes
- Redness
- Eyes may discharge a heavy sticky pus
- Eyes may feel gritty underneath the eyelids
- Upon waking you may find that your eyelids and lashes may stick together from the mucus that has dried on them overnight.

In babies:

- If their eyes are red or they appear to be itching them yet they are not producing tears.

- If conjunctivitis seems present in one eye.
- Call your doctor if you suspect your baby has conjunctivitis.

Causes

Many things besides **allergies** and **bacterial or viral infections** can cause conjunctivitis. The condition may also be brought on if you are very stressed and not eating well. In children conjunctivitis can follow a cold or sore throat, and in babies it can occur if the baby's tear ducts were not fully developed at birth, or if they were exposed to bacteria at or soon after birth. If you think your baby has conjunctivitis contact your doctor immediately.

Treatment

Treatment can usually be taken care of at home, unless the conjunctivitis goes on for 5 days without improvement. Keeping your eyes and hands clean is very important, as it will help prevent the infection from spreading to other family members who come into contact with you or the germs as conjunctivitis caused by infections are highly contagious.

To treat **viral or bacterial** conjunctivitis follow these steps:

- Keep your eyes clean, wash them often and if you use a cloth towel or washcloth, make sure nobody else will use it.
- Apply a **warm** compress for 5-10 minutes three or four times a day.
- Your doctor will likely prescribe **antibiotics** in the form of eye drops or ointments if the conjunctivitis is caused by a bacterial infection. **Antibiotics will not help in cases of viral infection**.

For **allergy** related conjunctivitis:

- Keep your eyes clean and flushed.
- Apply a **cool** compress for 5-10 minutes three or four times a day.

- You can ask your doctor about anti-allergy drugs that will help relieve the condition.

When to Call Your Doctor

- Your eye has been physically injured.
- The redness in your eye is affecting your vision.
- Your eyes become red while wearing contacts.
- The condition has not improved after a week.
- The person affected is a baby.

To Prevent the Spread of Conjunctivitis

- Wash your hands often, especially is the condition is caused by an infection.
- Do not touch the affected eye, and if you must, then wash hands immediately afterwards and do not touch other things so to avoid transferring the bacteria/virus.
- Do not share towels, face cloths, pillowcases, or anything else that might come into contact with the eyes. Change the items after each use, for example, if you have conjunctivitis, do not use the same towel over and over to clean your eyes; use it once and then use a different one.
- If your child contracts bacterial conjunctivitis (Pinkeye) keep them out of school for a few days to help avoid spreading it to other children.

Chapter 16

Corns and Calluses

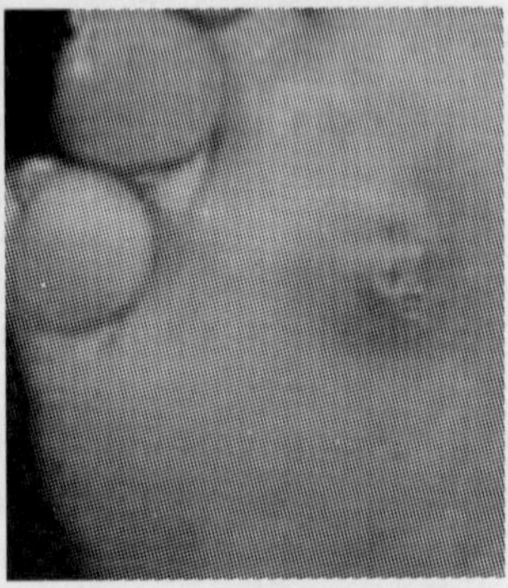

Corns and Calluses are the most common conditions of the skin on your feet. They can be found anywhere on the foot, but usually occur over bony areas. This happens because the pressure and stress on those areas is greater and dead skin forms and collects there forming corns and calluses. While these conditions are painful, they are usually easy to correct.

Classification

There are many different types of corns and calluses, named and classified by their location on the foot. The two conditions are close to the same thing, as both are caused by excessive rubbing on a part of the foot. The main difference is that corns are found on the tops and in between toes, while calluses are found on the outside of the foot. Common causes for the rubbing and extra stress in these areas is incorrect padding in shoes, flat feet, bone spurs, and hammertoes. On rare occasions calluses are caused by a sweat gland that has become blocked up with dead skin and the nerve going to the gland becomes affected. Listed below are some of the more common kinds of corns and calluses.

- When it is under the big toe joint it is called a *pinch callus*.
- When it is on an exposed part of the toe it is called a *hard corn*.
- When it is in between the toes it is called a *soft corn*.
- When it is found at the end of a toe it is called a *distal clavus*.
- Calluses are often found on the heels, a high stress area. These calluses are prone to crack and fissure, which may lead them to become infected. However they are easy to manage.

Treatment

Treatment of corns and calluses is easy, and the first thing you should do when they have developed is buy a better pair of shoes that will not rub in the same place. Shoes with a large toe box are recommended to avoiding corns and calluses in the toe area. Make sure you buy shoes that fit, avoid shoes that are too narrow or too wide. Low heeled shoes are also recommended for relieving pressure on the legions. Next you will want to get rid of the corns and calluses you have. Do NOT try to cut or burn off these legions! Home remedies, such as rubbing the area with a pumice stone, are effective, but they leave the skin rough and unsightly. Salicylic acid treatments can be dangerous. The paints and pastes may damage healthy skin as it removed the dead skin of the corn or callus, causing more damage, discomfort, and opening the body to infection. Here at Scivolutions we have come up with a way to remove corns and calluses and still keep you safe! The solution is our new corn and callus bandage kits. During the day you wear a special **Hydrocolloid** bandage over the affected area to soften the skin, keep it moist, and relieve some of the pain. At night, right before you go to sleep you apply a salicylic acid patch and foam covering to the area, cutting the acid patch to the needed size. At night your foot does not move around much, which means that the patch will stay in once place, and the acid will not affect the healthy skin around the corn or callus. This is the most effective and painless way to treat these painful problems. These pads SHOULD NOT be used by diabetics, people with poor circulation or blood supply, over open wounds or deep cuts, irritated or infected areas, on moles, warts, birthmarks, or (on or near) mucous membranes (mouth, nose, anus, genitals, lips, face). If after several days use pain and discomfort has not lessened, consult your doctor who may choose to remove the legion in a minor operation under local anesthesia.

Prevention

Corns and calluses are easy to prevent if you take the right steps.

- Do not wear shoes that are too tight or too loose. Both can cause rubbing that can lead to **blisters**, corns and calluses.
- If you find a certain part of your show is rubbing against your foot and causing discomfort place padding in the shoe or a bandage on your foot over where the rubbing is occurring. these help decrease friction and discomfort. In some cases you can bring the shoes to a shoemaker to have them try and stretch or fix the shoe so that it doesn't rub.
- Wearing thick socks with shoes can help absorb pressure, while tight socks or stockings leave you less protected.
- Change your walking style. If you notice that you tend to walk on the sides or your feet, or on your toes you're often more prone to developing blisters or corns and calluses in those areas because they're receiving more pressure. By learning you shift your weight better you can avoid these discomforts.

Chapter 17

Cardiopulmonary Resuscitation (CPR)

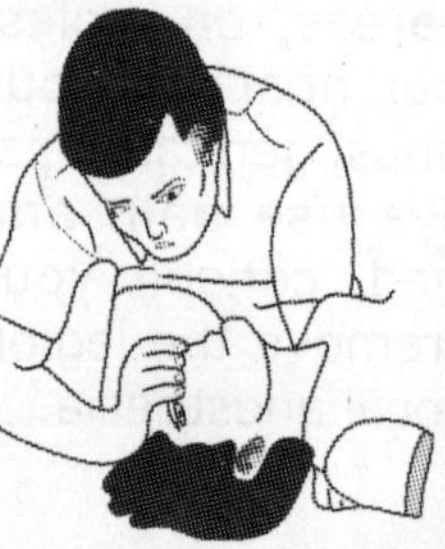

CPR is most commonly needed when someone goes into cardiac arrest (a heart attack) without notice, or they are choking on something and need assisted breathing. Below you'll find methods on how to deal with these situations until help arrives.

CPR for Adults

1. CALL

Check the victim for unresponsiveness. If there is no response, Call your doctor and return to the victim. In most locations the emergency dispatcher can assist you with CPR instructions.

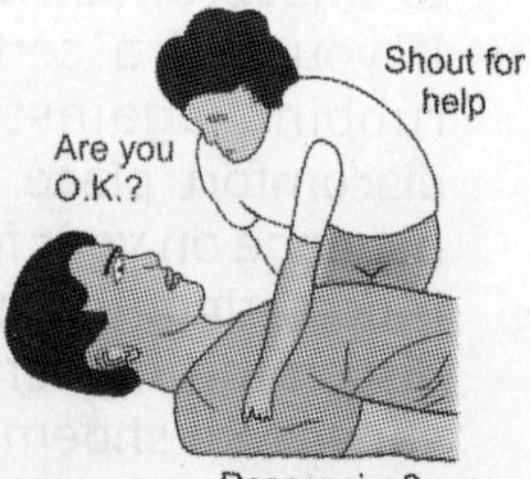

2. BLOW

Tilt the head back and listen for breathing. If not breathing normally cover the mouth with

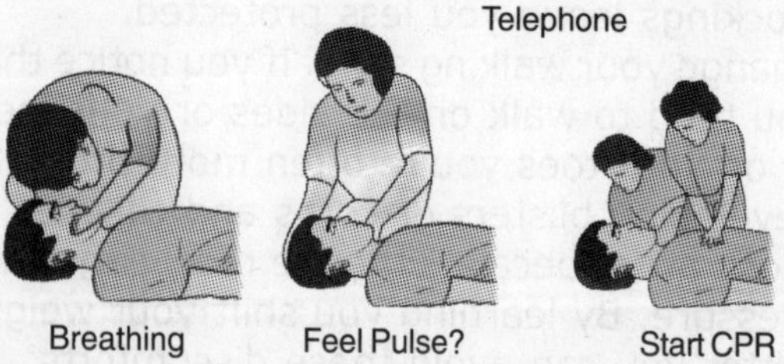

yours and blow until you see the chest rise. Give 2 breaths. Each breath should take 2 seconds.

3. PUMP

If the victim is still not breathing normally, coughing or moving, begin chest compressions. Push down on the chest 11/2 to 2 inches 15 times right between the nipples. Pump at the rate of 100/minute, faster than once per second.

CONTINUE WITH 2 BREATHS AND 15 PUMPS UNTIL HELP ARRIVES

NOTE: This ratio is the same for one-person and two-person CPR. In two-person CPR the person pumping the chest stops while the other gives mouth-to-mouth breathing.

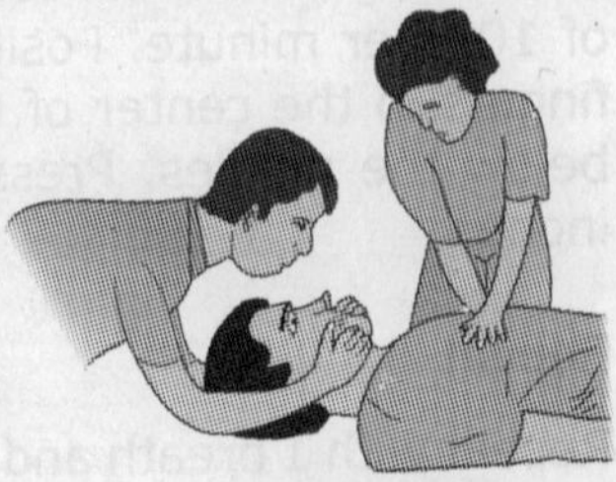

Mouth-to-mouth Breathing
Consider 2 rescuer CPR 1:5

CPR for Children (Ages 1-8)

CPR for children is similar to performing Quick CPR for adults. There are, however, 4 differences:

1. If you are alone with the child give one minute of CPR before calling your doctor.
2. Use the heel of one hand for chest compressions.
3. Press the sternum down 1 to 1.5 inches.
4. Give 1 full breath followed by 5 chest compressions.

CPR for Infants (Age <1)

Shout and Tap

Shout and gently tap the child on the shoulder. If there is no response, position the infant on his or her back.

Open the Airway

Open the airway using a head tilt lifting of chin. Do not tilt the head too far back.

Give 2 Breaths

If the baby is NOT breathing give 2 small gentle breaths. Cover the baby's mouth and nose with your mouth. Each breath should be 1.5 to 2 seconds long. You should see the baby's chest rise with each breath.

Give 5 Compressions

Give five gentle chest compressions at the rate of 100 per minute. Position your 3rd and 4th fingers in the center of the chest half an inch below the nipples. Press down only 1/2 to 1 inches.

Repeat

Repeat with 1 breath and 5 compressions. After one minute of repeated cycles call your doctor. If you feel a pulse return give one breath every 3 seconds and discontinue chest compressions.

What Complications Can Occur?

Vomiting is the most frequently encountered complication of CPR. If the victim starts to vomit, turn the head to the side and try to sweep out or wipe off the vomit. Continue with CPR.

The spread of infection from the victim to the rescuer is exceedingly rare. Most cardiac arrests occur in people's homes—relatives or friends will be the ones needing to do CPR. Even CPR performed on strangers has an exceedingly rare risk of infection. There is NO documentation of HIV or AIDS ever being transmitted via CPR.

Chapter 18

Dental Medicine

Dental Injuries

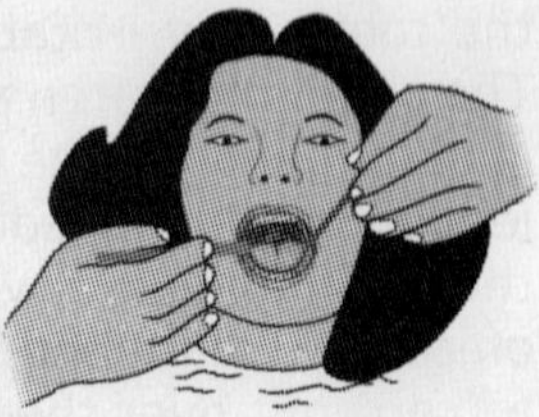

Dental injuries can be caused by a variety of facial traumas. Whether the injury is caused by making the save in the game or taking a spill from your bike, it's important to know how to take care of these injuries. Dental injuries involve not only the teeth, but the jaws, muscles, and gums around them. Most hospitals have oral surgeons who can handle emergency tooth removals and jaw fractions. If the injury has added head and neck trauma, go to the emergency room. Injuries like broken teeth or those knocked out of the mouth can be dealt with a dental office.

Dental Injury Classification

Tooth Fractures (chipped or broken teeth)

These fractures can range from minor to severe. Minor injuries involve chipping only the outer tooth layers while severe injuries involve vertical, diagonal, and horizontal fractures of the tooth root. The tooth is made up of three layers, the enamel, dentin, and the pulp. The enamel and dentin are the two outer protective layers of the tooth. The enamel is the white hard surface, and below that is the yellow layer of dentin. The innermost living part of the tooth is called the pulp. Because only 1/3 of the tooth is visible (known as the crown) in the mouth X-rays are necessary to determine the extent of the tooth fractures.

Chipped Teeth

These injuries are minor and involve only the enamel layer of the tooth. In these instances, the tooth is not out of place and the gums are not bleeding. The tooth may not be sensitive to temperature or food, but rough edges on the tooth may irritate the tongue and cheek. The pulp is not often at risk here and treatment is not urgent. On the way to the dentist, sugarless gum or orthopedic wax may be placed over the tooth to ease any discomfort. At the dental office, the treatment is usually a filling or having a "cap" put over the tooth to protect the pulp and restore normal tooth contour.

Fracture of Enamel and Dentin

This fracture is deeper and like a chipped tooth, the gums are not bleeding and tooth is still in place. However, these fractured teeth may be sensitive to food and cold temperatures. Prolonged exposure of this fracture could lead to bacteria attacking the dentin and eventually result in pulp death. Death of these tissues can lead to infection and abscess. Because of this, these injuries should be treated within days of the injury. An anesthetizing cream will be placed over the dentin, followed by a dental filling and cap will be placed over the tooth. A follow up X-ray will be required 3-6 months later to ensure that the pulp has not died.

If the fracture was deep enough to do actual damage to the pulp then either the dying tooth will have to be removed or a root canal will have to be performed. The root canal is designed to save the tooth from (a) serious infection and (b) having to be removed. The root canal removes all the dying pulp tissue and replaces it with inert material.

Serious Tooth Fracture

A serious fracture is one that exposes both the dentin and the pulp. And should be treated immediately. This tooth may be loose or out of place and the gums may bleed. To prevent the tooth from falling out the dentist may have to splint it by bonding it to the adjacent teeth while the bone and gums around it heal. Because the pulp is exposed in this injury, there is a high risk of pulp death; therefore, a root canal is often performed on the first visit for the injury. However is the dentist decides to splint the tooth then the tooth will need to be reevaluated in 2-4 weeks to see if a root canal is needed. After the procedure, a filling or crown is added and the splint is removed. The most severe tooth injuries are the ones that fall vertically, horizontally, and diagonally on the tooth roots. In many cases, this leaves the tooth very loose and extraction is needed. The hole is then filled with a removable plate that contains a false tooth. On rare occasions, teeth with horizontal fractures near the tip of the roots don't need to be extracted. However, the tooth is closely observed and x-rayed periodically to watch for signs of infection and pulp death, in which a case a root canal would be needed.

Teeth Knocked Out

As many parents know, the upper two front teeth are the two most likely to be knocked out. Those who play sports are at a great risk of this, as are children who have protruding front teeth that have not yet been put into correct alignment.

In most cases, if a child's baby teeth are knocked out nothing is done because the teeth will be replaced with permanent teeth in time. Knocked out permanent teeth are different stories. These teeth should be retrieved and kept moist and clean (rinse in clean water or milk) and put back in their sockets as soon as possible. Time is the most important factor here. The soon a tooth is re-implanted the better chance it has to become reattached. Teeth re-implanted within an hour frequently reattach themselves. This can usually be done without the help of a dentist, but if you are at all unsure store the tooth in milk or clean water and brought to the dentist as soon as possible. Or if the victim is an adult or calm child, the tooth can be held within the cheeks inside the mouth.

After the tooth has been re-implanted, the dentist will splint the tooth for 2-8 weeks. This helps stabilize the tooth while the bone heals. During this time, the patient must take special care to eat mainly soft foods and brush all the other teeth to keep the mouth as clean as impossible to ward off bacteria. In adults, the re-implanted tooth should have a root canal performed in 1-4 weeks, but in children, however, this is often unnecessary because the roots may not have fully developed. These teeth are observed for 5 years to make sure the pulp is healthy and no root canal procedure will be needed.

For most re-implant patients over the counter medications like acetaminophen (Tylenol) or ibuprofen (Advil) are fine for pain relief. Chlorhexidine mouth rinse may be prescribed to prevent gum disease and inflammation, since splinted teeth cannot be brushed normally. The splint also usually collects added tartar and debris. Oral antibiotics and tetanus toxoid injections are considered for patients with lacerations on the gums and mouth.

Teeth Displaced

Often instead of being knocked out of the mouth, teeth are displaced. This gives the tooth the appearance of seeming longer, shorter, or "bent" to the side, front, or back. Luckily this injury isn't an emergency, but a trip to the dentist is recommended as the sooner the tooth is realigned the better (and faster) the tooth will become correctly realigned. Sometimes the trauma can cause injury to the pulp so the tooth is monitored for several months to determine if a root canal, or tooth extraction is required.

Prevention

Prevention for dental injuries is fairly basic. Braces align teeth properly and facemasks and mouth guards have been shown to reduce trauma to the teeth, gums, jawbones, and joints. Mouth guards reduce the deformation of the skull when a force is directed at the chin. Mouth guards reduce the deformation of the skull when a foce is directed at the chin. Mouth guards have become very important, almost eliminating the injuries that occurred to the face and mouth. While mouth guards can be purchased in stores the best ones are custom made by your dentist. The store bought mouth guards are less expensive, but are not made for the athelete and may become loose, uncomfortable, and make cause problems with speech or breathing. A well fitting mouth guard should do none of the above.

Chapter 19

Depression

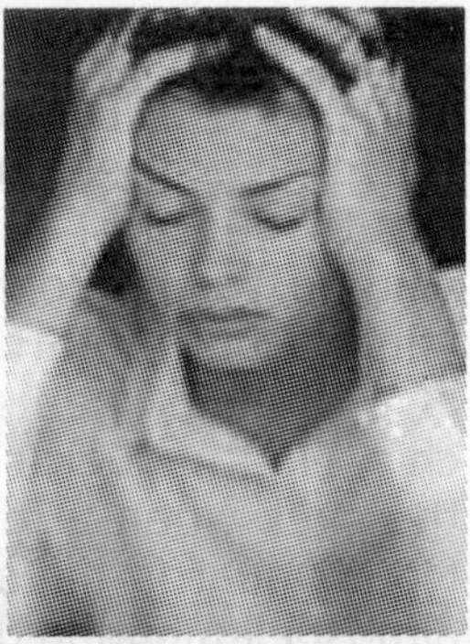

Millions of people (Indians) suffer from the disease, yet somehow to too many people the subject of depression is still considered to be relatively taboo and is not discussed as it should be. Depression is not just a bad case of "the blues", it's a very real and very serious illness. To those who would bypass treatment, or would look down upon seeking help and talking to a doctor, know this: ***The leading cause of suicide is untreated depression.*** Realize that depression can happen to anybody, no matter their age (including infants and the elderly), sex, ethnicity, race, economic standing etc. It is *never* something to be ashamed of.

Depression isn't just feeling sad, blue or "empty"; it's a chemical imbalance in your brain, it is not a character flaw or a sign of weakness. In some cases the imbalance is mild, and will right itself in time (time being a several months to a year). Other times it's severe and chronic and will take a lifetime of therapy, medicines, and other treatments. In either case, you do not want to leave the depression untreated. Ignoring the signs and feelings of depression is about as safe as ignoring a tingling in your left arm and pain in your chest, or a lump in your breast. You don't want to wait to see if it's a heart attack or cancer, because by then it's often too late, you would get help as soon as you started seeing the signs. If you have a friend who is losing a large amount of weight, looking pale, and complaining about being fat, you don't want to wait for them to collapse from malnutrition before telling them they need to get help. The same theory works with depression—it can be deadly if ignored. Sometimes people who suffer from depression can't see it, and it's important for the people who care about them to read the signs for them and get them help. In the following sections you'll find:

- Information of several of the different types of depression.
- Signs and symptoms.
- How to help.
- If depression becomes/threatens to become suicide, facts and symptoms, how to deal with it, what to say.

Classifying Depression

Although you should always leave diagnosing to the professionals, this section will give you a brief insight into several of the different types of depression. It should be noted that each type varies in severity and duration and that symptoms differ from person to person.

Dysthymia: This a chronic but mild form of depression. People who suffer from this are not unable to function, as in some other forms, but may function in a slower less than "full steam" fashion. They may not take pleasure in many things that a person usually would, and may often "feel bad". Those with Dysthymia are also prone to major depression episodes although not everyone will have them. This is one of the most prevalent forms of depression.

Major Depression (Unipolar Depression): Another very prevalent illness, major depression affects about 9.9 million Americans per year, (It is also nearly twice as common in women as in men). People suffering from major depression will have times when they feel perfectly normal, and then other times when they feel depressed, sad, slowed down, and in "a fog". This illness can be disabling as it tends to affect sleeping habits, appetite, physical health, mood, behavior and ways of thinking. If you've already experienced one episode of this type of depression then you have a better than half chance of having another during your life time. This for of depression, like all the others has a wide range of mild to serious and short term episodes to long term. Left untreated episodes commonly last around 6 months to a year, however if you leave major depression untreated you run the risk that it will lead to suicide. stressing the point, if you think you or a friend may be suffering from any type of depression mild or not, go talk to someone. They can help you determine if it is depression and then help you take the necessary steps to cure the illness.

Bipolar Depression (Manic Depression): There are two forms of this disease. And they are the last of the three most common depressive illnesses.

Bipolar I: A person with this form of bipolar disease will likely have dramatic mod swings ranging from severe lows (depression) to severe highs (mania).

Bipolar II: A person in suffering from this form will have milder manias (hypomania), and the lows will be of varying severity.

Mania vs hypomania: When a person is going through a manic phase they're likely to be very energetic and talkative, they may appear restless and like they're unable to slow down. They're prone to grandiose ideas and ideas, impaired or poor judgment and oftentimes embarrassing social behavior. They may also exhibit increased irritability and increased sexual desire. A person who has hypomania phases will also be very talkative and social, but instead of having slightly over the top ways of thinking, their minds are often extraordinarily sharp and clear and they're also more creative. They will feel as though they are in a fabulous mood until they fall back into a depressive period.

Cyclothymia: This is another form of a bipolar disease, but this one is a real mess. Moods are very unpredictable and can be up one day and down the next, the periods can go for days, weeks, or months at a time and periods where the person feels normal and few and far between. The manic part of the cycle is usually a Hypomania, and the depressive stage is usually mild.

SAD (Seasonal Affective Disorder): This is a disorder that follows a defined pattern, it recurs every winter. It's brought on by a persons reaction to the amount of light they receive. Since they days are shorter in the wintertime people are exposed to less light. Some symptoms of this disorder are low energy, sleepiness, larger appetite and over eating. It can often be helped by something known as photo therapy- which is morning exposure to bright full spectrum light. Photo therapy will help ease symptoms but is not a cure for the disease. A professional should again be seen if you suspect you are suffering from this.

Atypical Depression: This is not considered to be an official diagnostic category, but it is relatively common, so we will discuss it here. With atypical depression a person may feel happy and experience pleasure if the opportunity presents itself, such as a night out with friends, but the feeling is often short lived and soon replaced with feelings of heaviness, fatigue, increased appetite, and lack of motivation and energy until the next opportunity to have an enjoyable time presents itself. Other signs are moodiness accompanied by at least two of the following: overeating, over sleeping, extreme fatigue and rejection sensitivity.

Endogenous Depression: Depression can sometimes over take a person even when there has been no particular bad event, stressful situation, or apparent outside cause for the feelings of sadness and depression to be triggered. Luckily this form of depression often responds well to medication. you may wish to note that some doctors do not se this as a useful diagnostic category.

Post Partum Depression: This is a very common form of depression present in women who have just had a baby. Usually the feelings and symptoms of the blues are mild, but if they seem worse than mild, or last for longer than a few days help should be sought as this condition can be harmful to both mother and child.

Signs and Symptoms of Depression

Please realize that not all the symptoms will be present, and sometimes only one or two will be present. Make use of this list, use it as a checklist for yourself, or use it to try and evaluate whether your friend may be suffering from depression. If doing this for a friend, be very honest and answer how you think they would answer. Remember that everyone experiences some of these from time to time, and that is normal, it's when they begin to impact your life in a negative fashion and last 2 weeks or longer, when you want to seek help to find out what's wrong. Realize that there is no set number or combination of symptoms that mean you are suffering from depression. Also understand that many of these symptoms will appear gradually and may not be easy to recognize. If you're on medication for something else the medication may be causing you to feel this way, so make sure you talk with your doctor! NEVER be afraid to ask for help if you think you may be becoming depressed.

- I feel sad.
- I don't really feel sad, just "empty".
- I feel like I'm in a "fog".
- I feel so alone.
- Sometimes I feel like I don't "feel" anything.
- I feel like crying more often than usual.
- Sometimes I react in a big way to something I know is not a big deal—it feels like my emotions are out of control.
- I don't react the way I used to.
- I don't feel like "me".
- I don't like myself.
- I feel self-conscious.
- I don't have any confidence in myself, or have low self esteem.
- I feel worthless.
- I feel like there's no hope in this or other situations.
- I feel helpless.
- I feel like my life is going nowhere.
- I can't concentrate.
- I have a difficult time remembering things.
- I don't like making decisions.
- I can't think straight, like my brain isn't working right.
- I'm so disorganized, it feels like my head is spinning.
- I don't feel like talking anymore-I don't have anything to say.
- I feel guilty.
- I get angry a lot—almost like I'm going to explode.
- My thinking always seems to be negative.
- I'm more irritable.
- I have low tolerance.
- I get frustrated with everything and everyone.
- Sometimes I feel scared, but I don't know why?
- I feel "different" from everyone else.
- Occasionally, my heart will pound very hard and, I can't catch my breath, I feel tingly, my vision seems strange, and I feel like I

might pass out. It passes in seconds, but I'm afraid it will happen again. (This is a panic attack, these happen due to anxiety).

- I feel dizzy often.
- I have headaches, stomachaches, backaches, and/or pain in my arms and legs. Sometimes medicine doesn't seem to work.
- My vision seems blurred or "slow" sometimes.
- My whole body seems slowed down, speech, motion, thought, everything!
- I'm always tired, no matter how much sleep I get?
- I cannot fall asleep.
- If I'm sleeping and wake up, I cannot get back to sleep—even if I'm tired and it's the middle of the night.
- I don't feel like eating anymore.
- I'm always hungry and/or eating.
- I've lost or gained a significant amount of weight.
- I don't feel like taking care of my appearance or myself.
- I don't have fun anymore.
- I'm not really interested in activities I used to enjoy.
- I don't feel like going out with friends anymore.
- I'm afraid to call and ask friends to do things unless they call me first—I don't want to be rejected.
- I used to enjoy it, but now I'm not really interested in having sex.
- I'm always restless and jittery, like I can't sit still.
- I'm always getting into trouble.
- I use drugs or alcohol to escape or hide feelings.
- Sometimes I do things that are dangerous, or could hurt me.
- Sometimes I intentionally hurt myself.
- Sometimes I feel like I can't go on living.
- I smile, but inside I feel terrible.
- Nothing I do makes me feel better.

- I've thought about, or attempted ***suicide.***
- In the wintertime, I always feel "down" and depressed.

How to Help

Whether you or someone you know is depressed it's important to recognize the disease for what it is, because the person suffering may not be able to. When someone is depressed it is often difficult for them to realize that they can get help, that things can get better and that they can be happy again. With children realize that depressive illnesses can be genetic and the sometimes children are born with the chemical imbalance and the signs are hard to read since they've always been there above. ***If you think, for any reason that your friend may be suicidal get help IMMEDIATELY if not sooner.*** The article below offers some straight forward information for friends and family of someone who is suffering from depression. Reiterating what the author says, this information is based on dealing with people who have been diagnosed with depression by a professional.

If You Know Someone Who's Depressed

This page assumes that the depressed person has been diagnosed and is in treatment.

Main Problems for Friends and Family

Let me start by saying that I, for one, appreciate your wishing to understand someone else's depression. I commend you for taking an interest in a very difficult subject and for wishing to help. In an indirect way, you're a victim of depression too because this illness impinges on everyone around the people who have it.

Pardon my bluntness, but there are a few things you really need to know, before you get too far into this subject.

1. You cannot cure someone else's *clinical depression.* It is not just sadness which can be waved off with a few kind words. It goes far deeper than that. If you are going into this with the heroic notion that you can somehow "fix" it for your friend, spouse or relative, then you need to disavow it immediately. Operating on this assumption will only frustrate you and does no one any good.
2. There are ups and downs in *depression recovery*. It is neither swift, nor steady. Your friend or relative is going to go on the decline, now and then. Don't think it's because you are failing them or they are not trying hard enough. The "roller-coaster" effect is just a part and parcel of depression.
3. Please don't tell a depression patient that "you understand." Unless you, yourself, have experienced clinical depression, you don't. And your friend, spouse or relative knows it. It's not a bad thing; since understanding depression means having it. I'd rather that no one, anywhere, understood it. The point here is to be honest with your friend or relative and don't profess things that aren't so. Sincerity will help him or her a great deal; it will engender trust, which every depression patient has a problem with, at one time or another.
4. No one wants to make your life miserable by being depressed. Try not to view someone else's depression as your own affliction. Rather, be grateful that you don't have clinical depression and try to realize what the other person is going through. Don't take the things your friend, spouse or relative says/does, personally. They aren't meant that way.
5. Recovery from depression is not just a matter of *taking anti-depressant medi-*

cation and *going to therapy.* Both the depression and recovery from it can totally change a person's life. Treatment involves a lot of fundamental changes in a person. At times, you'll wonder if it's the same person you've known for so long. Believe me, it is—the depression probably hid the "real person" from your view, up to the point that he or she was diagnosed and began treatment.

6. At times, it may seem that the person is actually pushing you away. This is very likely true. Most depression patients believe that they unduly affect those around them and will do anything to prevent that from happening. Thus, they isolate themselves from others. This kind of self-sabotage is actually a symptom of the illness itself. Don't let it overcome your relationship. Try to understand that this is often involuntary and irrational, and act accordingly.

Treatment

Therapy and medication, which will help cure you? One, the other, both? Studies have shown that talk therapy (as well as behavioral and interpersonal therapy) has been helpful, but in many cases can not fully fix the problem, just alleviate some of the symptoms. The studies continue to show that the best way to effectively treat depression is a combination of medication and therapy. However, it is also advised that you do not jump for the medications if you don't need them, and it should be seriously discussed with your doctor before you decide whether or not to take any. Realize that once you are on medication the battle isn't over. You've got to do some work to make yourself feel better because the medicine can't really do it or be as effective without some help from you. Remember that there are many people who care and are more than willing to help you find ways of dealing with this problem. There are also other alternative ways of dealing with depression. To learn more about them visit some of the sites at the bottom of this page. Never be afraid to ask for help.

It should also be noted that if you do not have insurance but are depressed or suicidal you can still go to your local emergency room and get help, as well as contacting the many depression and suicide support and help groups.

**A note on medication*: Medication is not for everyone and it affects everyone differently. A medicine that worked for a friend may make you feel worse. If you're put on a medication and after adjusting to it (this in many cases takes at least a month-consult your doctor.) and you are feeling worse than you did before, or if you're experiencing negative behavioral (or other) changes -becoming moodier, more irritable, lethargic, etc-consult your doctor they may decide to change your medication and put you on something different. Remember the medication is supposed to make you feel better and help alleviate symptoms, if your medicine isn't doing this then you need to contact your doctor.

Depression and Suicide

For friends and family. *Please understand that just because a person is on the road to rec*overy does not mean they will stay there. The road is a bumpy one, full of ups and downs and it's not uncommon for people to fall off now and again. Please be very aware of this. Depression can shut off the survival instinct (or at least temporarily block) in our minds. Because of this people who are depressed look at suicide differently that those who have just reached a crisis point and are not depressed. Depression victims give less warning, plan less and are often willing to resort to more desperate and painful measures. If they are not suicidal they may take up self injury and mutilation instead. This to them is a way to numb the pain on the inside by causing pain on the outside. These are things that can happen to anybody who is suffering from depression, no matter how unlikely a person they might seem to be to think of doing such a thing. Depression changes the way you think, and the way you react. If for any reason at all you think someone may be suicidal or causing injury to themselves get help NOW. Do not wait, do not finish reading this paragraph, just get help right now. Please realize that sometimes, even with the best help, medical care, love, and effort people will still follow through with suicide.

Chapter 20

Diabetic

Classification

There are two different categories of emergencies when it comes to diabetes. Hypoglycemia (low blood sugar) and Hyperglycemia (high blood sugar). Below is a little information and some signs and symptoms of each.

Hyperglycemia

Hyperglycemia (high blood sugar)- onset of this condition is usually slower, and may occur when the diabetic consumes a large amount of sugar when they are remotely inactive. It may also be a sign of ketoacidosis.

- Hot dry skin.
- Extreme thirst, or excessive thirst.
- Frequent need to urinate.
- Smell of acetone (nail polish remover) on the persons breath.
- Drowsiness.
- Unconsciousness, which may lead into diabetic coma if untreated.
- Blurred vision.

Treatment for Hyperglycemia

1. Do not give the person something sweet to eat or drink as it will raise their blood sugar even more.
2. Do not give the person an insulin shot. If the person is conscious and able, allow them to give themselves a shot. If they ask, you may give assistance.

3. Call a your doctor or bring the person to the ER if blood sugar is abnormally high, or if person is unconscious.
4. If help is delayed, give the person sugar free liquids.

Hypoglycemia

Hypoglycemia (low blood sugar)-the onset of this imbalance is usually rapid, and commonly happens when the diabetic is physically active and are not doing enough to maintain their sugar levels.

- Pale skin.
- Weak and tired.
- Confused (may act drunk).
- Aggressive or cranky.
- Hungry.
- Excessive sweating.
- Rapid pulse.
- May go to sleep and become unconscious.
- Seizure.

Treatment for Hypoglycemia

1. A diabetic should always try to carry something sweet with them, be it a non-diet soda, fruit, or some candy in case they go 'low'. Administering this sweet drink or food item will help reverse the effects of hypoglycemia and raise the persons' blood sugar levels. Glucose tabs and gels are available in most drugstores. Only give food or drink if the person is conscious.
2. If the person loses consciousness or cannot swallow then medical assistance is needed. Call your doctor immediately or take the person to the ER.
3. If the person goes into a ***seizure*** call your doctor immediately.
4. There is an injectable medication called glucagon, which is available by prescription. A family member or friend should learn how and where to administer this shot, which raises the blood sugar quickly.

Chapter 21

Drug Overdoses

When someone overdoses, speed is the most important factor, even more so than the substance that was overdosed on. This is because the longer someone goes without treatment, the more the drug is absorbed, and the more damage is done. People can die from drug overdoses.

Symptoms

When someone has OD'd they may be:

- Unconscious
- Seizing
- Confused
- Fainting, dizzy, uncoordinated, or drowsy
- Slow or rapid pulse
- Vomiting
- Acting strangely, drunk, psychotic, overly friendly etc.
- Have difficulty breathing
- Slurred speech
- High or low temperature
- Enlarged or extra small pupils
- Reddish face and heavy sweating
- Delusions or hallucinations.

Treatment

- Contact the poison control center and your doctor immediately.
- If the victim is unconscious check vital signs. If you need to, begin *CPR*.

- If the person is unconscious check the airways and clear them out (remove any pills, vomit, etc.).
- Once the unconscious person is 'stable' place them in the recovery position (lying on their side) and wait for help to arrive while keeping a close eye on them.
- If you find pills, syringes, medications, bottles and containers (from medications or drugs) or drugs around the person save them and give them to the medics when they arrive. If available save a sample of the vomit as well.
- If the person is conscious ask them what happened and most importantly keep them as awake and alert as possible.
- DO NOT try to induce vomiting unless instructed to do so by a medical professional. The poison control center will tell you what to give and how much to give based on the persons age/weight and other stats.
- DO NOT give the person anything to eat or drink unless instructed.
- DO NOT leave the person alone.
- Try to figure out the time when the drug was taken and what quantity was taken.

Drugs and Symptoms Chart

A list is given in next page of substances and the symptoms that overdosing on them will bring about.

Name	Examples	Signs and symptoms of over dosage
Acetaminophen	Tylenol®; Parafon forte®.	Nausea; vomiting; pallor; sweating; kidney failure; jaundice; difficulty breathing; delirium; and unconsciousness.
Alcohol	Beers; wines; spirits.	Changes of mood; lack of coordination; slurred speech; sweating; rapid pulse; vomiting; drowsiness; and unconsciousness.
Amphetamines	Benzedrine®; Dexedrine®; Methedrine®.	Excitement; dilated pupils; talkativeness; insomnia; tremors; exaggerated reflexes; bad breath; vomiting; diarrhea; fever; irregular, rapid heart rate; hallucinations; delirium; convulsions; and unconsciousness.
Anticoagulants	Dicumarol®; Coumadin®; Panwarfarin®:	Nosebleeds; pallor; bleeding gums; bruising; blood in the urine and feces; shock; and coma.
Antidepressants	(1) tricyclic compoundsóTofranil®; Elavil®.	(1) Dry mouth; dilated pupils; vomiting; irregular heart rate; retention of urine; hallucinations; lack of coordination; exaggerated reflexes; agitation; convulsions; unconsciousness; and hypertension.

Contd.

Contd.

	(2) MAO inhibitorsóNardil®; Parnate®.	(2) Agitation;hallucinations; exaggerated reflexes; irregular heart rate; sweating; retention of urine; convulsions; and muscular rigidity.
Antihistamines	Tripelennamine; diphenhydramine; chlorpheniramine, promethazine.	Excitement or depression; drowsiness; headache; irregular heart rate; nervousness; disorientation; lack of coordination; high fever; hallucinations; fixed, dilated pupils; delirium; convulsions; and coma.
Atropine	Hyoscyamine; scopolamine; stramamine.	Dry mouth; hot, dry skin; flushing; high fever; dilated pupils; irregular heart rate; excitement; confusion; convulsions; delirium; and unconsciousness.
Barbiturates	Amytal®; Nembutal®; Seconal®; phenobarbital.	Drowsiness; headache; confusion; lack of coordina-; tion slurred speech; lack of reflexes; slow breathing rate; and coma.
Benzodiazepines	Librium®; Valium®; Mogadon®; Xanax®.	Drowsiness; dizziness; lack of coordination; and, in rare cases, coma.
Caffeine	Coffee; tea; No-Doz®; APC.	Restlessness; excitement; frequent urination; rapid pulse; nausea; vomiting; fever; tremors; delirium; convulsions; and coma.

Contd.

Contd.

Cannabis	Hashish; marijuana.	Overdose usually causes only sleepiness.
Chloral hydrate	Noctec®; Somnos®.	An overdose of chloral hydrate produces symptoms similar to a barbiturate overdose, but chloral hydrate may also cause vomiting.
Cocaine	Cocaine; crack.	Stimulation followed by depression; nausea; vomiting; anxiety; hallucinations; sweating; difficulty breathing; convulsions; cardiovascular collapse; severe hypertension.
Contraceptive pill		Overdose may cause nausea and vomiting. It does not usually require emergency medical aid, but it is advisable to consult a physician.
Digitalis	Lanoxin®; Crystodigin®; Purodigin®.	Vomiting; excessive salivation; diarrhea; drowsiness; confusion; irregular heart rate; delirium; hallucinations; and unconsciousness.
Diuretics	Hygroton®; Lasix®; Dyazide®.	Massive urine output and irregular heart rate. Rarely there may also be skin rashes and abnormal sensitivity to light.
Glutethimide	Doriden®.	Drowsiness; lack of reflexes; pupil dilation; slow breathing rate; and coma.

Contd.

Contd.

Hallucinogens	LSD; psilocybin; mescaline; phencyclidine (PCP).	The symptoms of an overdose are not always readily distinguishable from the normal effects of these drugs, which vary betweeen individuals. The effects include hallucinations; nausea; confusion; and lack of coordination. In some cases, especially with PCP, there maybe paranoia; delusions; extreme anxiety; aggressive and violent behavior; depression; seizures; coma; cerebral hemmorrhage; and even death.
Ipecacuanha	Ipecac syrup.	Nausea; vomiting, sometimes blood-stained; diarrhea; abdominal cramps; irregular heart rate; and cardiac arrest.
Iron	Iron supplement tablets and syrup.	Nausea; vomiting, sometimes bloodstained; abdominal pain; pallor; headache; confusion; convulsions; and unconsciousness.
Narcotics	Opium; heroin; morphine; Methadone®; codeine.	Pinpoint pupils; drowsiness; shallow breathing; muscular relaxation; coma; slow pulse and respiratory arrest.

Contd.

Contd.

Phenothiazines	Chlorpromazine; prochlorperazine; trifluoperazine.	Sleepiness; dry mouth; lack of coordination; muscular rigidity; tremors; uncontrollable facial grimacing; low body temperature; irregular heart rate; convulsions; and coma.
Quinine	Antimalarial drugs.	Vomiting; deafness; blurred vision; dilated pupils; headache; dizziness; rapid breathing; irregular heart rate; and unconsciousness.
Rauwolfia alkaloids	Reserpine.	Flushing; dry mouth; abdominal cramps; diarrhea; irregular heart rate; tremors; muscular rigidity; and unconsciousness.
Salicylates	Aspirin and many aspirin-containing painkillers.	Abdominal pain; nausea; vomiting; restlessness; noises in the ears; deafness; deep, rapid breathing; fever; sweating; irritability; confusion; delirium; convulsions; and coma.

Chapter 22

Ear Infections

Ear infections are notorious for several reasons- it's the most commonly reported diagnosis among children and it's also the most common cause for hearing loss among children. Ear infections, or otitis media, are the result of an infected and inflamed middle ear. It can occur in one ear or both and any hearing loss can be healed completely if acted upon promptly. These infections are most common during the winter and spring months, so parents should be especially watchful at this time if their child is showing any signs on an infection.

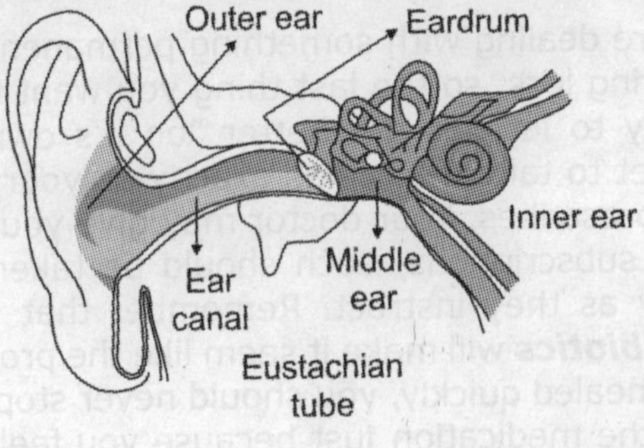

Ear infections, common as they may be, can be very damaging. Hearing loss, especially in children may impair learning capacity and in some cases slow speech development. Again, if treated promptly permanent hearing loss can almost always be avoided. Another reason these infections should be regarded as serious is that the infection can spread to nearby structures in the head.

Symptoms

Infants and Toddlers

- Pulling or scratching at ear (usually accompanied by several of the following)
- Hearing problems
- Ear drainage
- **Fever**
- Crying
- Irritability
- **Vomiting.**

In Children and Adults

- Hearing problems
- Earache
- Ear drainage
- Fever
- Dizziness
- A feeling of 'pressure' around/in the ears
- Vomiting and nausea.

Treatment

You're dealing with something permanent like hearing loss, so the last thing you want to do is try to let this get better "on it's own" or forget to take medicines exactly as your doctor prescribes. Your doctor may give you several subscriptions, each should be taken exactly as they instruct. Remember that while ***antibiotics*** will make it seem like the problem has healed quickly, you should never stop taking the medication just because you feel better, always take the full dosage given to you by the doctor unless instructed to do otherwise. Your doctor may also give you some questions about your medications.

Eye Injuries

Eye injuries can happen to anyone, and are quite common. Below are several types of injuries and suggested treatments.

Particle of Dust or Speck of Dirt in the Eye

- Do not rub your eye, as it may cause scratc-hing and other injury to your cornea.
- Gently lift your upper eyelid down over your lower one, allowing your eye to flush the particle of dirt out. Hold your eyelid like this for a minute or so or until you feel the object has been removed. This may be repeated as necessary.
- Blink your eye several times to help remove the object.
- You may also try to flush it out of your eye using a little bit of cool clean water (this may be more effective for dust, smoke, and heat burn to the eyes as opposed to dirt particles).
- Try not to remove it with your fingers as you may do damage to your eye.
- If object remains in the eye, keep it closed and go see your doctor.

If Something has become Embedded in the Eye

- Cover both eyes with a clean sterile pad and go to the doctors.
- Do Not try to remove the object or touch the eye.

A Hit or Blow to the Eye

- Quickly apply a cold compress to the area around the eye, not the eye itself, for about 15 minutes. This will reduce pain and swelling.
- A black eye or blurred vision may indicate eye damage and should be looked at by a doctor.

Cuts to the Eye or Eyelid

- Bandage the eye area gently with gauze and medical tape and get the person to the doctor as soon as possible.
- Do not attempt to remove any objects on the eye, or touch the eye.

- Do not apply pressure to the injured area, and do not rub the affected area.

Chemical Burns to the Eye

- Immediately flush the area with water, using your fingers to hold open your eyelids. Make certain that your fingers and clean and have no chemicals on them to avoid further damage and possible reactions. Continue to flush eye for at least 15 minutes. You may want to move your eye around while doing this to help assure the removal of all chemicals.
- Make sure the head is tilted so the chemicals and water do not flow into the unaffected eye.
- These burns should be looked at by a doctor as soon as possible to make sure no damage was done to the eye.

Prevention

Remember, eye injuries are usually preventable if the proper gear is worn. In labs always wear protective gear and goggles, and when playing sports make sure that you wear a mask or eye guard. When playing outside watch for branches and other things which might bring about an eye injury.

Chapter 23

Fainting

People most often faint when there isn't enough blood flowing to the brain. When this happens the person becomes unconscious, and the unconscious spell is usually brief. Fainting is not life threatening, although if the person faints on a regular basis it may be a sign of a more serious medical disorder, and should be discussed with your doctor. If a person feels faint (weak/lightheaded/dizzy/nauseous), have them lie down with their feet elevated above the level of their heart (about 8-12 inches), or have them sit with their head placed down between their knees.

Fainting May Occur Because of:

- Emotional and/or physical shock
- **Dehydration**
- Pain
- Overexertion
- Heart diseases
- Sudden changes in body position (most common in the elderly and pregnant)
- Insufficient fluid and food intake.

When someone faints there are many things that you need to check before beginning treatment for the fainting. Such as:

- Was the person injured when they fell? (**wounds**)
- Is the person showing any signs of **shock**
- Has the person had a recent head injury?
- Have they fainted recently?

- Are they pregnant?
- Are they breathing correctly/normally?
- Do they have a history of heart disease?
- Is the person properly fed and hydrated?

Treatment

- Lay the person on their back with their feet elevated above their heart, or 8-12 inches, if possible.
- Loosen any tight clothing and jewelry especially around their head and neck.
- Watch their airways, are they breathing correctly? If they stop breathing begin to administer **CPR.** If breathing stops then the situation becomes more serious and you should try to get medical help as soon as possible.
- Sometimes when people lose consciousness they vomit, you may want to turn the person onto their side in case this happens.
- If you suspect a head, neck, or spinal injury get medical help as soon as possible and do not move the person unless absolutely necessary.
- Do not try to give the person anything to eat or drink.
- If the person does not regain consciousness within 2 minutes call doctor or get other emergency medical help.
- If the person is older (over 40) contacting a doctor or calling doctor may be in order to make sure it was not a heart related problem.

Chapter 24

Your Family Disaster Kit

Why a Family Disaster Supplies Kit?

After a disaster, local officials and relief workers will be on the scene, but they cannot reach everyone immediately. You could get help in hours, or it may take days. Your family will cope best by preparing for disaster before it strikes. One way to prepare is by assembling a Disaster Supplies Kit. Store your kit in a convenient place known to all family members.

Place the supplies you'd most likely need for an evacuation in an easy-to-carry container. These supplies are listed with an*. Remember that disasters happen anytime and anywhere. And when disaster strikes, you may not have much time to respond. An earthquake, flood, winter storm, tornado, or other disaster could cut off basic services—gas, H_2O, electricity, phone—for days.

Water

Store water in plastic containers such as soft drink bottles. Avoid using containers that will decompose or break, such as milk cartons or glass bottles. A normally active person needs to drink at least two quarts of water each day. Hot environments and intense physical activity can double that amount. Children, nursing mothers and ill people will need more. Store one gallon of water per person per day (two quarts for drinking, two quarts for food preparation/sanitation).* Keep at least a three-day supply of water for each person in your household. Change your stored water supply every six months so it stays fresh.

Food

Store at least a three-day supply of non-perishable food. Select foods that require no refrigeration, preparation or cooking and little or no water. If you must heat food, pack a can of sterno. Select food items that are compact and lightweight. Canned juices, milk, soup (if powdered, store extra water) Rotate your stored food every six months. Keep items in air-tight plastic bags.

- Ready-to-eat canned meats, fruits and vegetables.
- Staples—sugar, salt, pepper.
- High energy foods—peanut butter, jelly, crackers, granola bars, trail mix.
- Foods for infants, elderly persons or persons on special diets.
- Comfort/stress foods—cookies, hard candy, sweetened cereals, lollipops, instant coffee, tea bags.

First aid, ask your physician or pharmacist about storing prescription medications.

Tools and Supplies

Keep the items that you would most likely need during an evacuation in an easy-to-carry container—suggested items are marked with an*. Possible containers include a large, covered trash container; a camping backpack; or a duffle bag.

- Mess kits, or paper cups, plates and plastic utensils*
- Emergency preparedness manual*
- Battery-operated radio and extra batteries* Replace batteries at least once a year
- Flashlight and extra batteries*
- Cash or traveler's checks, change*
- Nonelectric can opener, utility knife*
- Fire extinguisher: small canister, ABC type
- Tube tent
- Pliers
- Tape
- Strike anywhere, waterproof matches
- Aluminum foil

- Plastic storage containers
- Signal flare
- Paper, pencil
- Needles, thread
- Shut-off wrench, to turn off household gas and water
- Whistle
- Plastic sheeting
- Map of the area (for locating shelters).

Sanitation

- Toilet paper, towelettes*
- Soap, liquid detergent*
- Feminine supplies*/Personal hygiene items*
- Plastic garbage bags, ties (for personal sanitation uses)
- Plastic bucket with tight lid
- Disinfectant/Household chlorine bleach.

Clothing and Bedding

Include at least one complete change of clothing and footwear per person. Re-think your kit and family needs at least once a year, update clothes.

- Sturdy shoes or work boots*
- Hat and gloves
- Rain gear*
- Thermal underwear
- Blankets or sleeping bags*.

Special Items

Remember family members with special needs, such as infants and elderly or disabled persons.

For Baby:*

- Formula/Powdered milk
- Diapers
- Bottles
- Medications.

For Adults:*

- Prescription medications (heart medicines, insulin, antibiotics etc.).

- Contact lenses and supplies/Extra eye glasses.
- Entertainment—games and books.

Important Documents

Keep these records in a waterproof, portable container:

- Will, insurance policies, contracts, deeds, stocks and bonds.
- Passports, social security cards, immunization records.
- Bank account numbers/Credit card account numbers and companies.
- Inventory of valuable household goods, important telephone numbers.
- Family records (birth, marriage, death certificates).

Chapter 25

Fever

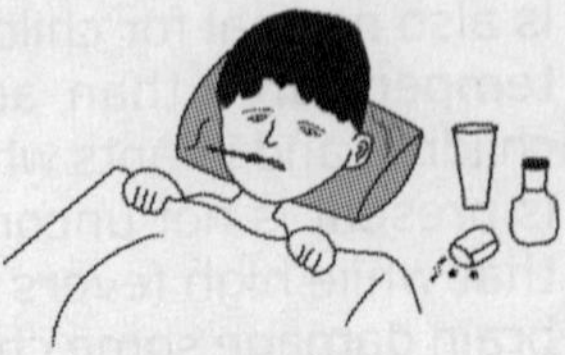

A fever is what happens when your body temperature rises higher than the average 98.6 degrees Fahrenheit (37 Centigrade). Fevers can be caused by many things, and range in severity from mild to potentially fatal. Some more common causes are:

- **Bacterial and viral infections** (colds, flu's, strep...).
- Sore and Strep throats.
- Urinary tract infections and inflammatory bowel disease.
- Earaches.
- **Shock.**
- Respiratory infections (tonsillitis, laryngitis, bronchitis).
- Some medications, such as those for high blood pressure, antibiotics, antihistamines etc. Ask your doctor if you think your medication may cause fever.
- Mononucleosis (mono).
- More serious things like pneumonia, **meningitis**, appendicitis, tuberculosis, cancer, leukemia, AIDS and HIV.
- Hodgkin's disease and Non-Hodgkin's lymphoma.
- Rheumatoid diseases, and Juvenile rheumatoid arthritis.
- Heat related illnesses such as **heatstroke**.

It is also good to keep in mind that fever

may not always be caused by illness, but instead by normal everyday factors. Things like hot foods, excessive clothing layers, exercise, excitement and anxiety, and menstrual cycles in women can all raise the body temperature by several degrees. In the case of strenuous exercise the temperature may even go up as high as 107 degrees, which in older children and adults is ok if it only lasts a short while. It is also normal for children to have higher body temperatures than adults- so high fevers in children and infants when only a minor infection is present is not uncommon. It is good to note that while high fevers are not directly linked to brain damage some children may have a febrile **seizure** as a result of a fever which may cause brain damage.

Fevers that are 102 or under are considered low-grade and can be treated at home by drinking lots of fluids and resting.

If your fever is higher than 102 then it's considered a high-grade fever and your doctor should be notified.

Fevers also behave in different ways; sometimes they jump high quickly then drops down again (known as spiking) and other times they increase and decrease in a regular fashion (known as cyclic). Bouts of chills and shivers often accompany fevers, but the person should not be heavily bundled up in blankets as this will raise their body temperature further. Instead cover them lightly and administer some fever relief medicine (if the fever is heat induced, like heatstroke, DO NOT administer any medications).

Sometimes a fever just seems to appear and hang around for a few days or even a few weeks for no apparent reason. If this happens contact your doctor, this often happens because of a 'hidden' infection.

Treatment

Fevers can often be treated at home, even if a trip to the doctors is necessary. Here are a few things you can do to help ease the discomfort of the person suffering from the fever.

- Administer some fever reducing medicine, but make certain that if the person is a child under age 18 the medicine contains NO ASPIRIN. Also do not give any medication if fever is heat induced. If person is having a seizure or is unconscious, administer no medication and contact your doctor immediately.
- Allow the person to rest.
- Give them lots of fluids to drink, such as juice and warm tea with honey. If they feel nauseas give them some clear cool sweet soda like ginger ale.
- Give the person a bath in lukewarm water (about 98 degrees Fahrenheit) this will help cool them down a little. Do not use cold-water, it will add to their discomfort and will not be any more helpful than lukewarm water. Do not use rubbing alcohol as it's absorbed by the skin and may send the person into shock.
- If they have the chills, cover them lightly and administer fever-reducing medicine. Heavy blankets and hot drinks will cause their body temperature to rise higher.
- If they are suffering a fever induced by a heat related illness go for treatment.

Chapter 26

Food Poisoning

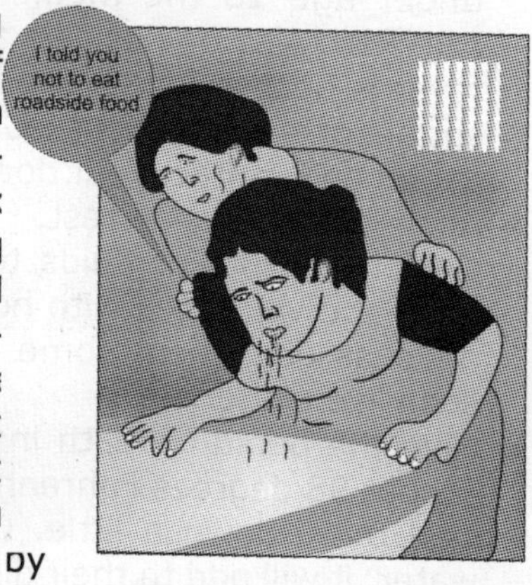

Food poisoning affects millions of people each year. Often people who think they're suffering from a case of the flu or a stomach bug are actually victims of a mild form of food poisoning. This illness is caused by viruses or bacteria that are found in food. Sometimes you get sick because the food is spoiled, and has gone bad, or because the food was not cooked correctly, or because a food touched some other food that was uncooked-such as if you have some uncooked chicken lying on a cutting board, and then cut some vegetables on the same cutting board without thoroughly cleaning it first.

Some common food poisoning culprits are listed below:

- *Salmonella and Campylobacter:* These bacteria are found in warm blooded animals, like poultry, cattle, pigs etc. The bacteria can be contracted from raw meat, undercooked poultry, raw/undercooked eggs, or un-pasteurized dairy products.
- *Clostridium perfringens:* You're privy to

catching these bacteria if you consume raw or undercooked meat, poultry, eggs, un-pasteurized dairy, for fish. If you have made a soup, gravy or stew with any of those products and it has been stored or refrigerated improperly for a few hours you are also at risk for contracting these bacteria.

- *Escherichia coli (E. coli):* These bacteria live in the healthy intestines of cattle, and are caught by consuming undercooked beef, especially ground beef–like in hamburgers– or in un-pasteurized milk.
- *Listeria:* These are associated with raw food that comes from animals.
- *Staphylococci:* These bacteria are different, they affect the human skin, nose and throat, and are transmitted when someone infected with it touches food.
- Shellfish-such as mussels, clams, oysters etc can also contain microorganisms that can make you sick-especially during red tide season.
- **Short incubation (ie, within 1 d, usually <16 h)**
  - Chemical causes (ultrashort incubation): The onset of nausea, vomiting, and cramps within 1-2 hours is observed in poisonings involving metal, fish-associated toxins (eg, scombroid, ciguatera), shellfish-associated toxins, monosodium glutamate, or mushrooms. The toxic agent in shellfish-and ciguatera-related disease is derived from dinoflagellate organisms present in the fish or shellfish. Note that neurologic symptoms can present weeks later. Amanita mushrooms can lead to hepatorenal failure.
  - Bacterial causes-Emetic syndrome (1-6 h)
    - S aureus*: Nausea and vomiting are caused by the action of preformed enterotoxins A-E.*
    - Bacillus cereus *(emetic syndrome, indistinguishable from staphylococcal food poisoning): This spore-forming rod*

is present in raw rice grains. The emetic toxin is a preformed heat-stable toxin produced upon germination of the spores.

– Bacterial causes-Diarrheal syndrome (8-16 h)
  - *B cereus* (diarrheal syndrome): The diarrheal toxin is a heat-labile toxin formed after sporulation.
  - *Clostridium perfringens* type A: Diarrhea and abdominal cramps occur within 1 day of ingestion of cooked meat stored at 15-60°C. Slow cooling allows heat-activated spores to germinate and to elaborate the enterotoxin.

- **Intermediate incubation (1-3 d)**
  - *Diarrheal disease:* This category comprises bacterial and viral infectious pathogens. The clinical presentation depends on the target organ (ie, small bowel or large bowel), which varies depending on the pathogen.
  - *Diarrheal disease, large bowel enteritis:* Fever and constitutional symptoms usually accompany the diarrhea caused by invasive pathogens in the large bowel. Dysentery, bloody stools with mucous, and cramps or tenesmus are typical.
    - Campylobacter jejuni*: This is a leading cause of bacterial food-borne illness in the United States. Vomiting is uncommon, and the illness is short and self-limiting.*
    - Shigella *species: Shigellae cause the prototypical diarrheal syndrome with blood, mucous, and pain that is termed bacillary dysentery. Tenesmus and small-volume stools are typical. Toxemia may be severe, occasionally causing seizures in children.*
    - Enteroinvasive *E coli* (EIEC): Several serotypes of diarrheagenic *E coli* possess *Shigella*-like invasiveness factors

that allow mucosal invasion. The disease is a febrile dysentery that mimics shigellosis.

- Salmonella *species, nontyphoidal salmonellosis: This is a zoonotic infection acquired from bovine or poultry reservoirs and is very common in the United States. The iilness can range from mild nonbloody diarrhea to a severe dysenteric illness.*
- Salmonella *species, enteric (typhoid) fever: Enteric fever occurs in travelers or recent immigrants and is a systemic toxic illness.* Salmonella typhi *has an exclusively human reservoir and is acquired either via ingestion of a large inoculum in food or contaminated water or from personal contact with a carrier.*
- Vibrio parahaemolyticus*: Although it is a common worldwide pathogen, in the United States,* V parahaemolyticus *infection is restricted geographically to the Atlantic and Gulf coasts. The diarrhea is profuse and watery, and blood is not commonly present in the stool.*

— Diarrheal disease, small bowel enteritis

- Enterotoxigenic *E coli* (ETEC): Enterotoxin-producing strains of *E coli* are the most common cause of traveler's diarrhea. The diagnosis is clinical; fever and bloody stools typically are absent.
- Vibrio cholerae *(01 and non-01 strains): Cholera is likely only in endemic areas and during epidemics. The profuse diarrhea and vomiting can lead to dehydration and prostration.*
- Viral agents (Norwalklike viruses, rotavirus, adenoviruses, astroviruses, caliciviruses): Vomiting and headache accompany the diarrhea and fever more commonly with viral than with bacterial infections.

    - All the large bowel pathogens also secrete enterotoxins that appear to cause profuse watery small bowel diarrhea in some patients.
  - Botulism: Nausea, vomiting, skeletal muscle paralysis, and autonomic symptoms occur within 18-36 hours of ingestion of food containing *Clostridium botulinum*. The disease is mediated by preformed toxin in older children and adults, but it may follow ingestion of spores in infants. Diarrhea occurs only in approximately 5% of patients; instead, constipation may be noted.
- **Long incubation (3-5 d)**
  - Enterohemorrhagic *E coli* (EHEC): Hemorrhagic colitis with a 5-10% risk of progression to HUS is observed in food-borne infection with bacterial pathogens that produce cytotoxins termed verotoxins or Shigalike toxins. *E coli* O157:H7 is one of many such cytotoxin-producing *E coli* strains that reside in the gut of cattle. Although these organisms can cause mild nonbloody diarrhea, hemorrhagic colitis is the usual symptom. Mild abdominal pain, malaise, and transient fever are followed by watery diarrhea. Bloody stools and more severe abdominal pain ensue 3-4 days later. When HUS occurs, its onset is 2-4 days later.
  - Yersinia *species*
    - Yersinia enterocolitica *most often causes a febrile illness with abdominal pain due to mesenteric lymphadenitis in which diarrhea is not prominent. The illness can mimic appendicitis. The illness may be prolonged, lasting 2-3 weeks. In infants, a diarrheal illness is common, with occasional septicemia. The diagnosis is made with blood and stool cultures. Treatment is indicated only for infants with septicemia.*

  - Yersinia pseudotuberculosis: *The symptom complex for this uncommon infection includes fever, rash (scarlatiniform or erythema nodosum), and abdominal pain.*
- **Very long incubation (1-4 wk)**
  - This category comprises parasitic FBDs, but shorter incubation periods can occur, especially in *Entamoeba histolytica* infection.
  - Parasitic
    - Giardiasis: The spectrum of illness ranges from asymptomatic carriage to acute watery diarrhea, but a subacute intermittent diarrheal illness also is common.
    - Amebiasis: *E histolytica* is a protozoan that causes dysentery and extraintestinal, most commonly hepatic, abscesses.
    - Cryptosporidiosis: The organism *Cryptosporidium parvum* causes a diarrheal illness with fever and abdominal pain.
    - Cyclosporiasis: Frequent watery stools, which can be accompanied by fever and a relapsing course, characterize this FBD caused by *Cyclospora cayetanensis*.
    - Trichinosis is a rare illness, caused by *Trichinella spiralis,* that is acquired by ingestion of contaminated or raw pork, bear, or moose meat. Gastrointestinal tract symptoms are followed by muscle inflammation and periorbital edema.
    - Cysticercosis: This infection is caused by the larval stage of pork tapeworm and most often is acquired by ingestion of food or water contaminated with the ova of the tapeworm rather than from eating raw pork.
    - Anisakiasis, fish tapeworm, and flatworm infections: These uncommon worm infestations occur after consumption of certain types of raw fish.

- — Bacterial
  - ▪ Listeriosis: Diarrhea in *Listeria monocytogenes* infection may be mild, but systemic symptoms are prominent. The diarrhea has a short incubation period (<48 h), but symptoms of systemic spread appear weeks later. The major risk is that of maternal infection during pregnancy. Neonatal sepsis and meningitis follow amniotic fluid infection. Older children and adults can develop meningitis. The infection is a particular hazard to individuals who are immunocompromised.
  - ▪ Brucellosis: This is a febrile illness now only rarely acquired in the United States. The food source is raw or unpasteurized milk or cheese, most commonly from goats (*Brucella melitensis*).
- — Viral: The incubation period of hepatitis A is 15-50 days for this viral hepatitis transmitted via the fecal-oral route.
- — Protozoal, toxoplasmosis: A febrile and subacute lymphadenitis results from ingestion of undercooked meat. A nonspecific illness with systemic symptoms and generalized lymphadenopathy can occur in healthy individuals, or an asymptomatic infection can result. Persons who are immunocompromised can develop CNS infection.

• Type of food consumed: The following is a checklist of commonly implicated food items that may suggest the etiology of a FBD:
- — Tap water when traveling abroad
- — Undercooked eggs, egg salad, or egg-containing salad dressings
- — Shellfish, including mussels, oysters, or scallops
- — Wild mushrooms
- — Fish (specify type)
  - ▪ Ciguatera—Grouper, red snapper, barracuda, or amberjack

  - Scombroid—Tuna, bluefin tuna, skipjack, mackerel, marlin, mahi mahi, or puffer fish
- — Raw fish prepared at home (sashimi or sushi, especially Alaskan salmon, rockfish)
- — Chinese food
- — Meat (specify if undercooked or wild game)
- — Unpasteurized milk, cheese, eggnog, ice cream, or juices
- — Cream pastries or cookie and cake batters
- — Home-canned goods
- — Food in corroded metal containers
- — Fresh produce, including fruit
- — Hot dogs, deli meats, or chitterlings (ie, pork innards)
- — Soft cheeses or cheese sauces
- — Tofu
- — Rewarmed rice

- Travel or activity
  - — Farming
  - — Pet contact
  - — Daycare
  - — Foreign travel, especially coastal
  - — Gulf coast of the United States
  - — Camping
  - — Group picnic or family reunion.

Symptoms

Symptoms of food poisoning often mimic gastroenteritis and stomach flus, except that the symptoms will appear suddenly and often within several hours of eating the contaminated food. Here are some common symptoms.

- Abdominal cramps
- Abdominal gas
- **Nausea and vomiting**
- Watery or bloody diarrhea
- **Fever**
- **Headaches**.

Treatment

Treat food poisoning much like you would treat a case of gastroenteritis-replace lost fluids and give medication to control any vomiting or feelings of nausea. In more severe cases hospitalization may be required. Remember that while most cases of food poisoning are mild, it can be fatal and should always be taken seriously.

Prevention

- Keep your hands clean! Before handling any food, after using the restroom, coughing, sneezing, smoking etc.
- When it comes to preparing foods, make sure the surfaces you're preparing on are clean, and wash your hands in between handling different meats and poultry and other produce.
- Wooded surfaces are not good for meats, poultry, and fish, as they aren't as easy to sanitize as plastic ones. It is suggested that you have two cutting boards, one specifically for vegetables, fruits and other foods that don't need preparation (such as deli meats or cheeses) and another exclusively for meats, poultry, and fish. Keep these surfaces especially clean.
- Wash all produce before cooking or preparing.
- Wash all cooking utensils and surfaces thoroughly after each use.
- Cook beef, poultry, eggs and fish thoroughly before eating.
- Try not to eat or drink any undercooked foods containing eggs, un-pasteurized dairy, poultry, fish or beef. Keep cooked and prepared foods away from uncooked foods to avoid cross contamination.
- People who should take special care are young children, the elderly, pregnant women, and those who have a chronic illness or an already weak immune system.

Chapter 27

Haemorrhoid (Piles)

What are Haemorrhoid?

Haemorrhoid (often known as Piles) are masses of tissues present in the anal canal. Surrounded by muscle and elastic fibres, these clumps contain blood vessels. Most people think that Haemorrhoid are abnormalities in the anus. The reality is that Haemorrhoid are present in all human beings irrespective of age, sex and race. They are a part of the normal anatomy and physiology within the anal canal.

But sometimes the haemorrhoidal cushions enlarge and cause symptoms of pain, itching or bleeding. This is the abnormal or diseased haemorrhoidal activity. The extent of haemorrhoidal abnormalities may vary from individual to individual.

In its normal state, haemorrhoidal tissues act as a sort of gatekeeper (or valve) of the anus and prevent unwanted leakages. They help in keeping the "gate" closed when you do not want it opened. Remember the times when you felt the urge to relieve (with no toilet in sight!) and clenched your butt muscles to stop the excreta from spilling over! The haemorrhoidal tissues did all the work and helped in keeping the anal gate clenched. These tissues also help prevent unwanted leakages during instances of coughs, sneezing etc. In the abnormal state haemorrhoidal tissues become enlarged and normal functioning is hampered causing discomfort to the affected individual.

Haemorrhoidal has been in existence for eons, in fact it is as old as mankind. However the incidence of Haemorrhoid is growing due to rapid changes in lifestyle and dietary habits.

The incidence of abnormal Haemorrhoid is the maximum in men and women of the age group of 45 - 65 years. Many factors can lead to affected haemorrhoidal tissues. These include pregnancy, diarrhea, constipation, hereditary causes, diet etc. This is explained in more detail in our section on causes.

The embarrassment associated with Haemorrhoid has ensured that the problem is kept under wraps. After all discussing your haemorrhoidal problems with another person is not a very appealing thought.

If you suspect that you have Haemorrhoid it is important that you gather as much information as possible and be well informed about this condition. The best thing to do is to visit a doctor for a correct diagnosis of the problem and to rule out other causes for the bleeding. In many cases lifestyle changes have helped redress the condition. In some cases, off-the-shelf medicines and herbal remedies have also proved to be extremely helpful.

Symptoms of Haemorrhoid?

The most common symptoms of Haemorrhoid are :

- Pain around the anus and lower bowel when you are relieving yourself (opening bowels)
- Itching around the anus area
- Discharge of mucus (a slimy liquid)
- Bleeding around the anal area. Blood is generally not mixed with excreta but is present around the anus. The blood discharged is usually bright red in color. You may observe it while using toilet paper.

- A feeling of something hanging or a bulge/ lump at the anus.
- A feeling of a full rectum. Feels as though your bowels are not completely emptied.

Causes of Hemorrhoids

Due to the extra stress in the lower part of the rectum/anus which leads to bleeding, and can be prevented by reducing anal stress and providing protection/treatment to mucus membrane of intestine, this brings relaxation to the body.

There are a group of muscles around the opening of the anus which help in passing stool. These muscles are called the anal sphincter. The stool collects in the rectum and the sphincter muscles keep the anus closed. When the pressure from the stool increases on the walls of the rectum, the sphincter relaxes and stool is pushed out of the anus.

Pressure is needed to expel the excreta through the anus, but sometimes if too much pressure is applied (say during constipation) then that causes the hemorrhoids to enlarge and they may get pushed out of their normal position with the stool. This excess pressure could be caused due to any of the following reasons:

- Pregnancy
- Heavy Lifting
- Chronic Diarrhea
- Varicose veins
- Constipation
- Hereditary
- Obesity
- Uncomfortable seats

How are Hemorrhoids treated?

Hemorrhoids usually have a tendency to keep reoccurring, therefore most people feel that it is usually best to treat them as little as possible. In many cases, the problem usually disappears on its own, in a few days, even without any treatment. However this may not always be the case and if you have been suffering from piles for a long time then you know that it can be quite a nuisance. In this chapter we deal with some of the treatments available for hemorrhoids. These range from simple medications and over-the-counter creams to non-surgical and surgical procedures for dealing with piles.

Medications

If your hemorrhoids are not too troublesome or if the symptoms are very mild, then use medicated creams, or gels. All the creams are aimed at relieving itching and pain by reducing the swelling and bleeding from the piles. Some patients also find relief by applying cold compresses to the affected area. Even daily warm baths can help you deal with the pain and discomfort. If the medication is only a topical cream, then it may be applied with your finger. At times the medicines may need to be inserted inside the anal canal for which there are instruments such as pile pipes, which have holes on the sides that dispense the medication inside your rectum.

Some of the most simple treatment for piles are:

Stool softeners. Since straining and constipation are the biggest factors in causing piles, these medicines such as Docusate sodium act by increasing the absorption of water and fat into the stool, which makes it soft. The soft stool is easy to pass and this reduces the excess pressure on the hemorrhoids.

Natural Hemorrhoids Treatment

Best results are often shown when one reverts to nature in foods and habits rather than treatments. There are a number of natural remedies and products available for treating hemorrhoids in the market today. Some are in the form of pills while others are creams or gels. These products are derived from naturally occurring herbs such as butcher's broom, horse chestnut, bilberry and so on. These herbs work by improving circulation around the anal region, which reduces pain and itching and prevents the piles from reappearing. The mode of treatment usually varies depending upon the cause, severity, and duration of the disease.

Some foods that help in treating Hemorrhoids

There is a high correlation between hard-constipated stools and the occurrence of hemorrhoids. As has been explained earlier, the hard stools put too much strain on the anal region, which causes the hemorrhoidal tissues to protrude and enlarge. Keeping the stool soft and easy to pass helps a lot in preventing painful episodes of piles.

A diet rich in complex carbohydrates and fibre helps in preventing stools from getting too hard and constipated. Brocolli, Potatoes, Pasta, Wheat, Brown Rice and Blackberries are some of the leading sources of complex carbohydrates. Hemorrhoids occur more frequently in those patients who had a tendency to miss breakfast. That is because by missing a meal we rob our bodies of dietary fibre that helps in bulking up the stools. Similarly a diet rich in meat and dairy products also leads to constipation due to lack of fibre. Dietary fibre, especially insoluble fibre such as psyllium, is broken down slowly in the intestines. This gives the bacteria present in the walls of the intestines time to break down the fibre causing it to ferment. The extra fibre also absorbs water, which makes the stools soft and easy to pass. Most doctors recommend consuming atleast 20-30 grams of fibre per day.

Food products such as ground flaxseeds and oats are rich in fibre and help in making bowel functions regular. Prunes, which contain a gentle laxative substance called dihydroxylphenyl isatin also help in softening the stools. While consuming a high fibre diet, you should also drink atleast 6-8 glasses of water a day, because fibre binds well with water. Insoluble fibre can be obtained by eating Figs, Brown Rice, Dried Raisins and Currants, Wheat and Fresh Peas. Sometimes if too much fibre is added very suddenly in the diet, it may cause bloating and flatulence. But if you continue to consume the same quantity each day then the digestive system gets used to it. If you feel that the flatulence is too much then you can gradually increase the quantities in your diet. Raw vegetables can at times cause flatulence, but if they are slightly steamed before consumption then that problem does not occur.

If you suffer from constipation, try eating a few dried prunes or drinking some prune juice. In addition to adding fiber, prunes have a mild laxative effect.

Apart from the extra fibre and more water, a diet rich in vitamins and minerals also helps in treating hemorrhoids. Foods that contain vitamin C, zinc, anthocyanins and flavonoids, such as quercetin, are useful for patients with hemorrhoids. Flavonoids are particularly good for managing the symptoms of hemorrhoids as they help in strengthening the hemorrhoidal veins. Flavanoids can be found in many food products. For instance buckwheat and apples contain a type of flavonoid called rutin. The white skin between the peel and meat of citrus, cayenne and other peppers, currants and parsley are rich in Bioflavonoids. Citrus foods contain flavonoids such as hesperidin and diosmin. Brocolli, Pomegranates, Soyabeans, Tomatoes, Onions, Carrots and Blueberries are some of the other sources of flavanoids. Quercetin is found in Green Cabbage, White Grapefruit, Spinach, Grapes, Kale, Pears, Onions and Garlic. Vitamin C and Zinc help by promoting the healing process. Vitamin C can be found in foods such as Red Cabbage, Tangerines, Bell Peppers, Kiwi Fruit, while Zinc can be obtained by eating Barleym Chicken, Oysters, Wheat and Turkey.

Mega-Recipes

1. Spinach & Paneer over Brown Rice
2. Penne with White Beans, Carrots and Tomatoes
3. Roasted Sweet Potato, Apple and Onion Salad
4. Herb-Grilled Red Onions.

Chapter 28

Headaches

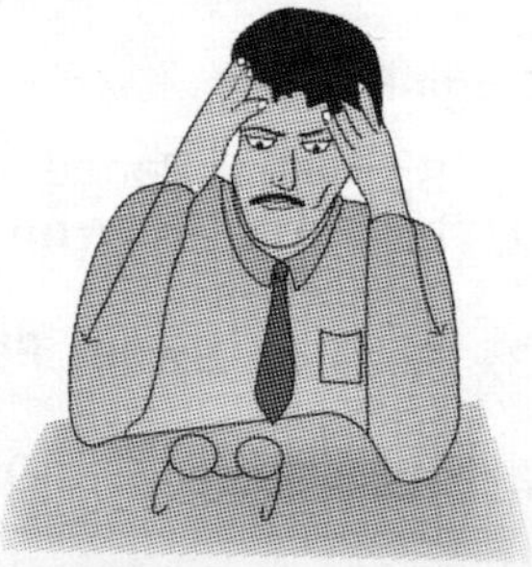

Headaches are a very common and troublesome occurrence and can be quite painful for the individual involved. Usually they are only minor health concerns, and can easily be treated with over the counter pain reducers such as ibuprofen or aspirin. However, if the headaches persist for days, are present with other symptoms and reoccur often you should consult your doctor to make certain there is no underlying problem. The two most common headaches are tension and sinus headaches. Sinus headaches are caused by things like **allergies**, head **colds**, and hay fever. Tension headaches are usually brought on by stress, excessive noise, poor posture, too much caffeine, eyestrain the grinding and clenching of teeth at night, and added tension in the scalp and neck muscles. Both of these can be treated with over the counter pain medication. Migraines are much more serious headaches.

OK, you have a headache, which one do you have?

- A dull, steady pain that feels like a band tightening around your head, you have a **tension headache**. These headaches are often accompanied by pain in the neck and shoulders as well.
- A steady pain in the area behind your face

that gets worse if you bend forward and is accompanied by congestion, you have a **sinus headache.**

- A throbbing pain around one red, watery eye, with nasal congestion on that side of your face, you have a **cluster headache**.
- Throbbing begins on one side, and causes nausea, you have a **migraine**.

Treatment

As mentioned before both sinus and tension headaches can be treated with mild pain killers, although for some sinus headaches—which usually accompany colds or allergies—your doctor may recommend a decongestant or antibiotic (the antibiotic is not being prescribed for the headache, but for the sinus infection that's causing the headache) instead.

Other simple ways to help relieve pain are to drink a cup or herbal tea (chamomile, lemon etc), take a nap, or (for tension or migraine headaches) gently massage your face with your fingertips. Do this by gently massaging your temples with a circular motion; repeat in the hollows at the sides of your eyes (by your nose), behind your ears, and over your neck.

When to Seek Further Professional Advice

- A severe headache is accompanied by vomiting or other severe symptoms.
- After a head injury, you are drowsy, with dizziness and other symptoms.

Chapter 29

Heart Attack

What is a heart attack?

The heart is a vital organ that pumps blood to various parts of the body. The heart receives oxygen rich blood through blood vessels called the coronary arteries. If these blood vessels become blocked, then the muscle of the heart does not get its supply of blood and dies. This is called a heart attack. The seriousness of the heart attack depends on the extent of damage to the heart muscle. The dead muscle may adversely affect the functioning of the heart by weakening the pumping effect, leading to (congestive heart failure), a condition which results in breathlessness and sweating of the feet.

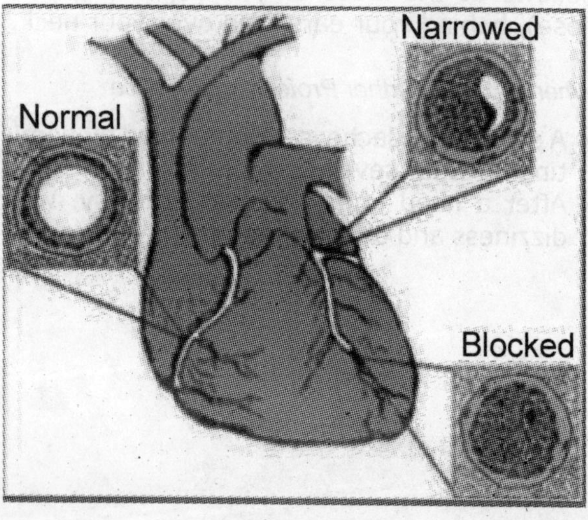

Why does it occur?

As we grow older, cholesterol deposits inside the blood vessels in various parts of the body, including the coronary arteries causing gradual blockage of blood flow. This gradual narrowing is called atherosclerosis.

Men are more likely to have a heart attack than women. The women are protected possibly by the influence of the female sex hormones, oestrogen and progesterone. These protective influences stay at least till menopause.

Asians, including Indians appear to be at a higher risk of developing a heart attack.

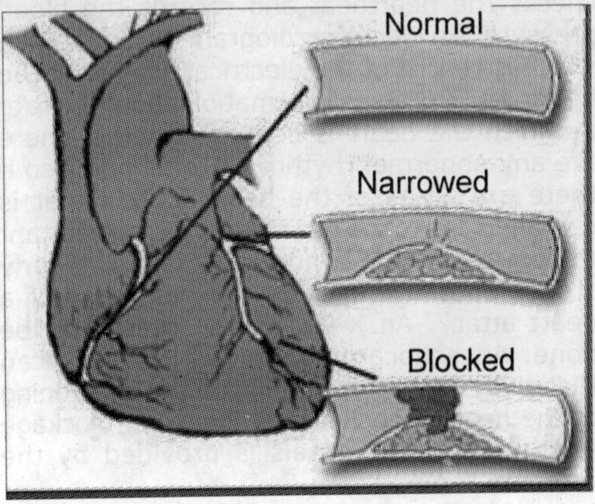

The risk factors include:

- Cigarette smoking
- Diabetes
- High blood pressure
- Overweight
- High cholesterol, and lower values of HDL v the good cholesterol
- Lack of physical activity

- A family history of heart attacks
- Stress, chronic anger and anxiety

What are the symptoms?

The signs may be difficult to identify and may mimic other conditions. Typically there is pain in the chest with tightness and difficulty in breathing. Sweating, nausea and feeling faint may be other symptoms. The pain may be in the front of the chest or behind the breastbone. From there it may go to the neck or left arm. In severe cases, the patient may look pale due to a fall in blood pressure rapidly leading to death.

How is it diagnosed?

The doctor takes a detailed medical history, checks the heartbeat and records the blood pressure. An electrocardiogram, ECG, is taken which is record of the electrical activity of the heart. An ECG gives information about the rate at which the heart is beating, whether there are any abnormal rhythm patterns and also if there are areas of the heart muscle that is damaged due to the heart attack. It is important to remember that a normal ECG in the early stages does not exclude the possibility of a heart attack. An X-Ray of the chest may be done. An echocardiogram is a type of scan that gives useful information on the functioning of the heart. Conclusive evidence of blockage in the coronary vessels is provided by the coronary angiogram.

What first aid should be given to a patient during an attack?

Prompt treatment of heart attacks can save lives. Till expert medical help arrives, the patient must be made to lie down and all tight clothing loosened. If an oxygen cylinder is available, the patient must be given oxygen. If nitroglycerine or sorbitrate tablets are available, one or two tablets may be put under the tongue. Aspirin should also be given in a soluble form.

What is the treatment?

Heart attacks require immediate medical attention and hospitalisation. The first few minutes and hours are critical. In the early stages, medicines can be given to dissolve the clot in the coronary arteries. The heart rhythm is monitored and abnormal rhythms are promptly treated. Pain relieving medicines are given and the patient is encouraged to rest and sleep. If the blood pressure is high, drugs are given to lower the pressure.

The exact treatment is individualised and depends on the patient's age and the severity of attack, the extent of damage to the heart and the extent of blockage in the vessels. Many times a more definitive procedure to remove the blockage may be necessary. This may be in the form of coronary angioplasty, dilatation of vessels using a balloon, or coronary bypass surgery.

How can heart attacks be prevented?

Those at high risk of developing heart attacks must take the following preventive measures:

- Their diet must be healthy and low in fats and salt, high in fiber and complex carbohydrates.
- Weight reduction is necessary for those who are over weight
- Physical exercise must be done regularly.
- Smoking must be stopped completely.

Those with diabetes, high blood pressure or high cholesterol must take drugs to keep their condition under control. Aspirin in low doses, in the long term, helps to prevent heart attacks and strokes, by thinning the blood and making it less liable to clot easily.

Chapter 30

Heat Illnesses

Heat illnesses are a common and treatable summer hazard. A heat related illness should never be ignored; if it is then the victim's condition will worsen and could lead to death. Heat illnesses can happen to anyone, but babies under a year old, the elderly, the sick, the physically active, and people exposed to hot weather conditions are at the greatest risk.

Dehydration

Dehydration is easier to prevent than treat. Your body, under normal conditions, has a certain balance of fluids and electrolytes. When this balance is disturbed other systems are affected and illnesses occur. Dehydration is a drop in fluid levels and can usually be treated easily with no lasting effects. Prevent dehydration by keeping your body hydrated. If you are doing something active outside such as hiking or a sport, you'll sweat and breathe a lot harder, losing more fluid than normal. Some medications also cause fluid loss. In situations like these, it's important to drink water or sports drinks (which replace electrolytes as well) whether you feel thirsty or not. If you feel thirsty, you're already showing signs of dehydration. It's good to know the symptoms of dehydration in case you are ever in a situation where you may be at risk. Below are some of the more common symptoms:

Early or Mild Dehydration

- Extreme thirst
- Flushed face
- Dry, warm skin
- Weakness
- Headache
- Dry mouth with thick saliva
- Decreased coordination
- Fatigue
- Smaller appetite
- Impaired judgment
- Dizziness that worsens as you stand and move
- Small amounts of dark yellow urine
- Arm and leg cramps
- Very few tears (when crying).

Moderate to Severe Dehydration

- Fainting
- Convulsions
- Low blood pressure
- Less sweating (internal cooling mechanism becomes ineffective)
- Severe arm, leg, stomach, and back cramps
- Bloated stomach
- Sunken 'dry' eyes
- Lack of skin elasticity (a bit of lifted skin takes longer to 'spring' back into place).

Dehydration Can Be Treated By

- Giving the victim more liquids than usual, but in small doses, too much at once could cause vomiting which would lead to even greater fluid loss. Water, sports drinks, and oral rehydration solutions (**ORS**) are best. Sports drinks and **ORS** replace both fluids and electrolytes. **ORS**'s can be bought or made. The drinks should be sipped slowly, in small amounts for about an hour. Even if you vomit while doing this, your body is retaining some of the fluids. Chilling the liquids can help, as it can prevent internal body temps from becoming to high and progressing to heat stroke.

- Nonprescription medicines that will help replenish fluid and electrolyte levels are available. Salt tabs however should be avoided, as they will lead to further dehydration.
- The person affected should be resting in the shade and should not resume activities until urination becomes normal (pale yellow and clear), and the other symptoms of dehydration disappear.
- Those suffering from dehydration have less of an appetite. If you fear you are becoming dehydrated (or want to avoid it altogether), make sure you eat and drink small amounts of food 5-7 times a day.
- In cases of severe dehydration, get the person to an emergency room, as untreated dehydration can lead to death.
- If a person who is severely dehydrated can drink, they should still be given the **ORS** and water.

Treatment and Symptoms of Heat Exhaustion

Heat Exhaustion

Heat exhaustion is similar to, and often follows, dehydration. It's what happens when you're losing more fluid and electrolytes than your body can handle. And although both fluids and electrolytes are being lost, exhaustion is a greater loss of electrolytes whereas dehydration is a greater loss in fluids. Heat exhaustion is a form of volume shock, in other words, the lack of fluid causes the blood vessels, especially in your arms and legs, to constrict. Luckily, this is a non-life threatening illness.

Symptoms

- Sweating
- Increased pulse and respiration
- Pale and clammy skin
- Fatigue

- Nausea and vomiting
- Slightly lowered or elevated temperature
- Exhaustion
- Lightheadedness and dizziness
- Possible heat cramps
- Feeling thirsty
- Decreased urine output.

Treatment

- With enough fluids and rest this illness is self correcting.
- A Sports drink or oral rehydration solution (**ORS**) should be given to replenish decreased electrolytes. Drink fluid slowly, as the body will absorb it better.
- Take a good long rest before continuing with your activities; if symptoms seem severe, you may want to see a medical professional.
- If the person is suffering from heat cramps a slightly salty drink (sports drink or **ORS**) and stretching the muscle should ease them. If they return, you should probably discontinue the activity you are doing for the rest of the day.
- If heat exhaustion is not properly treated, it may become Heat Stroke, which is deadly. If the person's temperature goes above 103° then treat them for heat stroke!

Prevention and Symptoms of Heat Stroke

Prevention

Keeping up with your body, is more important than keeping a fast pace with your friends. If you feel the symptoms of exhaustion coming on take a break, slow down, drink and eat a little before going on again. It will also be helpful to rest during the noontime hours, which are the hottest of the day. Wearing breathable clothing and a hat will also help to keep you cooler when taking part in physical activities on hot and humid days.

Heat Stroke

Heat stroke is a life-threatening emergency, and victims can die in just 30 minutes so help must be given quickly. Heat stroke is caused by an increase in the body temperature to about 104° (41°C). Temperatures over 105° can lead to death. This increase in temperature causes the brain to overheat. There are two types of heat stroke: fluid depleted (slow onset) and fluid intact (fast onset).

Fluid depleted (slow): The person has heat exhaustion, but continues to function in a situation. Eventually the lack of fluid will minimize the body's active heat loss capabilities to such an extent that the internal temperature will begin to rise.

Fluid intact (fast): The person is under extreme heat in a challenging situation, this overwhelms the body's active heat mechanisms even though fluid levels are sufficient.

Symptoms

- Hot and Red skin. Some victims will have hot dry skin (common in the elderly) and others will have hot wet skin (if, for example, they were previously suffering heat exhaustion) in all cases, however the skin should look red.
- Pale skin
- Pulse and respiratory rates increase
- Decreased urine output
- Argumentative
- Disoriented
- Increased temperature
- Combative
- Hallucinations
- Dilated and unresponsive pupils
- Seizures, which may lead to the person becoming comatose.

Treatment MUST Begin Immediately

- The most important thing to do is begin to lower the body temperature. Gently move the person to a shady or cooler spot and remove all non-cotton or un-breathable clothing. If possible, try moving the person to somewhere where medical assistance will be available. (Drive to the hospital, or a spot where an emergency team will be able to locate you and take over.)

- Pour cool (NOT cold) water over the person's extremities. If water is limited cool off the head and neck area first. Also, try fanning the person to increase air circulation and speed up sweat evaporation. If available place ice packs at the neck, armpits, and groin In That Order!
- While cooling the person off you should massage the extremities, which helps propel the cooled blood back into the persons core which will in turn lower their temperature.
- After their temperature has dropped to 102° then stop trying to cool them down, as hypothermia may begin and cause the person to shiver, which would generate more heat. Monitor them closely to make sure their temperature does not begin to rise again.
- If the person is able, begin to replace the fluids they have lost by giving them small sips of water or **ORS**. Sometimes, because they are temporarily mentally impaired it is impossible to get them to ingest fluids. In cases like that, continue the cooling process and try to get them to an emergency room.
- In more severe cases, CPR will need to be performed.
- Get the person to an emergency room as soon possible!! Your quick actions can save their life.

Heat stroke, like all other heat related illnesses is preventable by drinking an ample amount of fluids (not just water, as electrolytes will need to be replaced as well) when you are exposed to heat, or are being physically active. Remember, it is nearly impossible to drink too much water on hot days when you're active, and that your body absorbs it better when taken in in small amounts. It is also important not to rely solely on your body to tell you when you're thirsty as sometimes you become overwhelmed to quickly. So to stay safe drink often, not because you're thirsty but because you know you should.

Chapter 31

Herpes Zoster

What is Herpes zoster? What causes Herpes zoster?

Herpes zoster is a skin rash caused by the same virus that causes chickenpox. This virus is called the Varicella zoster virus (VZV) and is in the herpes family of viruses. After an individual has chickenpox, this virus lives dormant in the nervous system and is never fully cleared from the body. Under certain circumstances, such as emotional stress, immune deficiency (from AIDS or chemotherapy), or with cancer, the virus reactivates and causes Herpes zoster. In most cases of Herpes zoster, however, a cause for the reactivation of the virus is never found. Anyone who has ever had chickenpox is at risk for the development of Herpes zoster, although it occurs most commonly in people over the age of 60.

The herpes virus that causes Herpes zoster and chickenpox is not the same as the herpes viruses that causes genital herpes (which can be sexually transmitted) or herpes mouth sores.

What are Herpes zoster symptoms and signs? How long does Herpes zoster last?

Before a rash is visible, the patient may notice several days to a week of burning pain and sensitive skin. When the characteristic rash is not yet apparent, it may be difficult to determine the cause of the often severe pain. Herpes zoster rash starts as small blisters on a red base, with new blisters continuing to form for three to five days. The blisters follow the path of individual nerves that come out of the spinal cord in a specific "ray-like" distribution (called a dermatomal pattern) and appear in a band-like pattern on an area of skin. The entire path of the affected nerve may be involved, or there may be areas in the distribution of the nerve with blisters and areas without blisters. Generally, only one nerve level is involved. In a rare case, more than one nerve will be involved. Eventually, the blisters pop, and the area starts to ooze. The affected areas will then crust over and heal. The duration of the outbreak may take three to four weeks from start to finish. On occasion, the pain will be present but the blisters may never appear. This can be a very confusing cause of local pain.

Is Herpes zoster contagious?

Yes, Herpes zoster is contagious. Herpes zoster can be spread from an affected person to children or adults who have not had chickenpox. But instead of developing Herpes zoster, these people develop chickenpox. Once they have had chickenpox, people cannot catch Herpes zoster (or contract the virus) from someone else. Once infected, however, people have the potential to develop Herpes zoster later in life.

Herpes zoster is contagious to people who have not previously had chickenpox, as long as there are new blisters forming and old blisters healing. Similar to chickenpox, the time prior to healing or crusting of the blisters is the contagious stage of Herpes zoster. Once all of the blisters are crusted over, the virus can no longer be spread and Herpes zoster is no longer contagious.

What is the treatment for Herpes zoster? Should I visit my health-care professional?

There are several effective treatments for Herpes zoster. Drugs that fight viruses such as acyclovir, valacyclovir, or famciclovir, can reduce the severity and duration of the rash if started early (within 72 hours of the appearance of the rash). In addition to antiviral medications, pain medications may be needed for symptom control. Both nonsteroidal anti-inflammatory medications and narcotic pain control medications may be used for pain management in Herpes zoster.

The affected area should be kept clean. Bathing is permitted, and the area can be cleansed with soap and water. Cool compresses and anti-itching lotions, such as calamine lotion, may also provide relief.

What are the complications of Herpes zoster?

Generally, Herpes zoster heal well and problems are few. However, on occasion, the blisters can become infected with bacteria, causing cellulitis, a bacterial infection of the skin. If this occurs, the area will become reddened, warm, firm, and tender. You might notice red streaks forming around the wound. If you notice any of these symptoms, contact your health-care professional. Antibiotics can be used to treat these complications.

A more worrisome complication occurs when Herpes zoster affect the face, specifically the forehead and nose. In this situation, it is possible, although not likely, that Herpes zoster can affect the eye, leading to loss of vision. If you have Herpes zoster on your forehead or nose, your eyes should be evaluated by a health-care professional.

A rare complication of Herpes zoster is known as Ramsay Hunt syndrome. In this case, the cranial nerves (cranial nerves V, IX, and X) are involved. Symptoms may include peripheral facial nerve weakness and deafness. The typical rash is often observed around the ear and ear canal.

What is postherpetic neuralgia?

The most common complication of Herpes zoster is postherpetic neuralgia. This occurs when the nerve pain associated with Herpes zoster persists beyond one month, even after the rash is gone. It is a result of irritation of the nerves of sensation by the virus. The pain can be severe and debilitating. Postherpetic neuralgia occurs primarily in people over the age of 50 and affects 10%-15% of people with Herpes zoster. There is evidence that treating Herpes zoster with antiviral agents can reduce the duration and occurrence of postherpetic neuralgia.

The pain of postherpetic neuralgia can be reduced by a number of medications. Tricyclic antidepressant medications, as well as antiseizure medications, carbamazepine, pregabalin, have been used to relieve the pain associated with postherpetic neuralgia. Capsaicin cream, a derivative of hot chili peppers, can be used topically on the area after all the blisters have healed, to reduce the pain. Lidocaine pain patches applied directly to the skin can also be helpful in relieving nerve pains by numbing the nerves with local lidocaine anesthetic. These options should be discussed with your health-care professional.

Can Herpes zoster be prevented with a vaccine?

In May 2006, the U.S. Food and Drug Administration (FDA) approved the first vaccine for adult Herpes zoster. The vaccine, known as Zostavax, is approved for use in adults ages 60 and over who have had chickenpox. The Herpes zoster vaccine contains a booster dose of the chickenpox vaccine usually given to children. Tests over an initial four-year period showed that the vaccine significantly reduced the incidence of Herpes zoster in these older adults. The single-dose vaccine was shown to be more than 60% effective in reducing Herpes zoster symptoms and it reduced the incidence of postherpetic neuralgia by at least two-thirds. Studies are ongoing to evaluate the effectiveness of the vaccine over a longer term. People with weakened immune systems due to immune-suppressing medications, cancer treatment, HIV disease, or organ transplants should not receive the Herpes zoster vaccine because it contains live, weakened viral particles.

Since vaccination against VZV is now recommended for children, the incidence of chickenpox has been reduced. This is also expected to reduce the incidence of Herpes zoster in adults as these children age.

Herpes zoster At A Glance

- Herpes zoster is caused by the same virus that causes chickenpox and can be spread to people who have not had chickenpox.
- Herpes zoster, also known as herpes zoster, is not related to the sexually transmitted herpes virus disease called herpes genitalis.
- Herpes zoster may cause pain that can continue after the rash disappears.
- Steroids and antiviral drugs can help prevent long-term pain after Herpes zoster if they are started within the first two days of the appearance of the rash.
- A vaccine is available for people over 60 years of age to reduce the incidence and severity of Herpes zoster.

Chapter 32

Hydrocolloids

What Are They And How Do They Work?

Wouldn't it be great if you didn't have to worry about getting scars from your wounds and burns? Wouldn't it be great if you had hospital style dressings at home? Wouldn't it be great if you had a wound dressing the made the pain go away? What if I told you that this was all possible, and easy to obtain? All of the above are features of a Hydrocolloid. Dressings that, up until recently, were used only in hospitals for burns, minor wounds, and surgery patients.

Hydrocolloids are a thin dressing that is placed directly over the wound. Although it adheres to your skin, it will not adhere to the wound, which makes removal much less painful. The hydrocolloid is covered with a special absorbent material that absorbs fluid from the wound, and allows excess fluid to evaporate but at the same time is impermeable to oxygen, water, bacteria and other germs. In this way the hydrocolloid creates a moist humid wound environment, which promotes faster healing and helps prevent scarring. Because the wound is moist, no hard scab is formed. Hydrocolloids are the most natural way for the body to heal itself, and also the least damaging, as scabs leave scars and can be broken thus opening the body to new infection and damage.

When the dressing is applied to the wound the person will notice that almost immediately the pain will lessen or go away. The hydrocolloid can be left there for up to several days. If it falls off, it means that the wound has produced more fluid than the dressing could handle, and a new dressing is needed. When the dressing is removed, the wound itself and the new tissues being formed will not be disturbed, although a residue from the dressing may be left on the surrounding skin. This should be gently cleaned off before a new dressing is applied.

These dressings work best on wounds that are superficial granulated wounds that are releasing a low to medium amount of fluid. If you are bleeding heavily these dressing will not help you. If your wound needs a higher absorbency dressing you may want to try a hydrocolloid powder or paste, ask your doctor where you can find these and if they are right for your wound. If your wound has become *infected do NOT use these dressings!* Their safety has not yet been proven on clinically infected wounds!

In a study that involved laceration, abrasion and small operating incision patients, a hydrocolloid dressing was compared with a non-adherent dressing. The results were as follows. Although the healing time was the same for both groups, the patients using the hydrocolloids won out overall. Those using the hydrocolloids experienced less pain, and were able to carry out normal daily activities (such as bathing) without disturbing the wound or the dressings.

Chapter 33

Hypothermia

Hypothermia is a condition in which the body temperature drops below normal. This condition is brought on usually by staying in a cool place for an extended period of time. It is often a problem found in older people who may have other illnesses or be taking medications that interfere with their bodies ability to regulate temperature. Alcohol also has an effect on the body temperature. The usual temperature of the body is about 98.6°F (37°C), in cases of hypothermia the temperature drops below 96°F (35.5°C). It may not seem like a big difference but it can do severe damage to your body. Bad cases of hypothermia can cause an irregular heartbeat which in turn leads to heart failure and death.

What Should You Look For?

If someone claims they are unusually cold then take their temperature with a thermometer. Many oral thermometers will not record temperatures below what's just about normal. If no temperature can be determined try using a rectal or internal thermometer to get a more exact temperature. If no temperature shows up or it is below 96°F then call doctor for emergency help. You may have to keep a close eye on older people who may be reluctant to complain if they feel cold. If they do not state they are cold but you see some of the below signs you should take action:

- Confusion or sleepiness
- Slow, slurred speech

- Shallow breathing
- Excessive shivering or no shivering, stiffness in the arms or legs
- Poor control over body movements or slow reactions
- Weak pulse or low blood pressure
- Cold rooms, or signs that the person has been in a cold place
- A change in the way a person looks or behaves in cold weather.

Treatment and Recovery

The first and most important step is to make the person warm and dry. Those suffering from hypothermia must get medical help, but it's important to keep the person warm until help can be received. At the hospital the doctors will warm the body from the inside out, most likely by giving them warm fluids intravenously.

If help is not available, move the person to a warmer location, and if possible wrap them in a warm blanket to prevent further heat loss. Also try using your own body heat. Lie next to the victim but be gentle and do not handle them roughly. Rubbing the arms or legs to generate warmth may make the problem worse.

Recovery depends on the temperature your body drops to. If the temperature has not gone below 90 F (32.2°C) then the chance of total recovery is good. But if it falls in between 90 (32.2°C) and 80°F (26.6°C) then most people will recover but some permanent damage is likely. If the body temperature falls below 80°F then most victims will not recover.

Prevention

If you are on body temperature affecting medications, or you get cold easily don't let your home get too cool. If you are ill it is also important to keep the house warm enough that you don't make it worse. If you keep the house cool because of the price of heat, don't. Some states have programs to fund heating to protect against things like accidental hypothermia. If you have low income and don't use lots of money on heat contact your local power companies to talk about getting help. You could also "weatherize" your home by heating only the rooms that are used the most.

As mentioned before the elderly are often vulnerable to hypothermia and even in nursing homes they may be at risk. If the temperature is lowered too much, those who are sick or on medication may find it difficult to keep warm.

Another thing that is important to consider that many people overlook is the wind chill. Wind chill is the brisk wind that makes people loose heat faster. On some days the temperature may be fairly warm, but the wind chill could be low enough to make you stay indoors or dress warmly.

Some illnesses also make people more susceptible to hypothermia such as memory disorders, slow thyroid, or other hormonal disorders, strokes or other disorders that cause paralysis and reduce awareness. Severe arthritis, Parkinson's disease and others that limit activity and conditions that curb the normal blood flow can also cause problems. Medicines used to treat nausea, depression and anxiety, as well as some over the counter cold medicines also affect heat loss. Make sure to consult your doctor if you have any questions.

Chapter 34

Indigestion

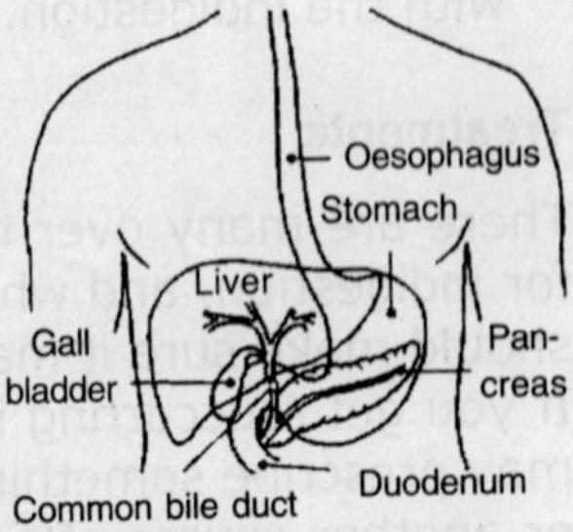

Indigestion is a common, usually harmless, discomfort that virtually everyone will feel at some point in his or her lifetime. Indigestion is the pain or sick feeling one occasionally experiences after eating. It is caused by:

- Over-eating.
- Eating too quickly, and not chewing enough
- Eating while stressed.
- Drinking excessive alcohol.
- Eating food that disagrees with you (ex: spicy foods make some people feel sick).
- Frequent use of pain relievers and other medications when taken without food.
- Chronic indigestion can also be brought on by smoking and obesity.

Signs of Indigestion Are:

- Heartburn.
- **Nausea** (mild to strong) or vomiting.
- Gas or burning.
- Abdominal pressure (bloating).
- Flatulence.

It is good to note that while indigestion is usually harmless it can be a symptom of a more serious problem. If you get indigestion daily, or suspect it may be a result of something more serious, consult your doctor. You should also consult a health professional if:

- Any abdominal pain continues for six hours or longer.
- You have repeated bouts of severe indigestion.
- Your indigestion always follows after you consume dairy products.
- You are experiencing other symptoms along with the indigestion.

Treatments

There are many over the counter treatments for indigestion, and when purchasing one you should make sure it matches your symptoms. If you get reoccurring indigestion your doctor may prescribe something else for you to take, or another course of action.

Prevention

You can also do things in your everyday life to help you avoid indigestion, for example, watch your weight, avoid over eating/drinking, chew slowly, and do not smoke. Avoiding fatty and highly spiced foods will help, as will eating fruits with digestive enzymes such as kiwi or pineapple. Also if you're a frequent gum chewer, give it a break and see if your indigestion ceases. Drinking tea may help to calm your stomach, however, add only a minimal amount of sugar. After eating take time to relax, drink lots of fluids during the day (hot lime-water is best) and fewer liquids during meal times.

Chapter 35

Influenza

Influenza- the Flu

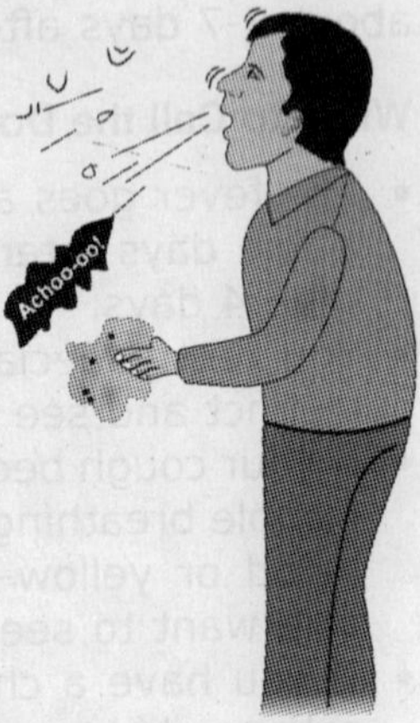

Every year in the India there are millions of people infected with the flu and about 20,000 flu related deaths. Luckily, we have ways to treat this illness; unluckily the virus changes every year. Because this happens and there are several strains going around at once, doctors can only select a few strains to make a vaccine from. To help immunize people from the virus, a flu shot must be taken every year. The flu spreads quickly and easily, via coughing or sneezing on your hands, or other things that people touch. The virus spends 1 to 4 days incubating before the symptoms arise.

Symptoms

- Coughing which may start dry and become more 'wet'. This cough may last for up to 2 weeks and in smokers it may lead to bronchitis and pneumonia.
- Chills and sweating.
- Nasal congestion (runny nose, stuffy nose).
- Tiredness and weakness (may last for a week or so even after the person has recovered).
- Sore throat.

- Vomiting and diarrhea in children 6 and younger.
- Loss of appetite.
- Muscle aches and pains, especially in the arms, legs and back.
- Fever of 101°F or more (up to 104/106°F). This fever can last for a day, or as long as a week.

If you have the flu you are contagious for about 5-7 days after the start of symptoms.

When to Call the Doctor

- The fever goes away and then comes back a few days later, or if it persists for more than 4 days.
- You feel especially concerned. Trust your instinct and see a doctor for advice.
- If your cough becomes wheezy, or you have trouble breathing. If you begin coughing up blood or yellow-green colored mucus you also want to see a doctor.
- If you have a chronic illness like diabetes, asthma, kidney, blood, heart, or lung problems.
- If you're suffering from severe confusion, seizures/convulsions, loss of consciousness, spasms, bleeding, heart irregularity, ear pain, or prolonged headache.

Risk

You are at High Risk for the Flu if:

- You're 50 or older.
- You work in a hospital or nursing home where you may be exposed to people with the virus.
- If you have a chronic illness (diabetes asthma, kidney, blood, heart, or lung problems).
- If you are taking medications that suppress your immune system. Such as medications for an organ transplant.
- You will be in your second or third trimester or pregnancy during flu season.

Your Children are At Risk if

- They have asthma or a chronic disease that affects their breathing, like cardiovascular disease.
- They are taking medications that suppress their immune systems.
- They are around people who are at high risk for catching the flu.
- They have sickle cell anemia, or Reye's syndrome.

Treatment

- Non-aspirin pain relievers may be given (Tylenol for children, ibuprofen for teens and adults) to help ease fever, muscle and headaches.
- Drink plenty of fluids to keep yourself hydrated and keep mucus and other fluids from getting too thick and increasing breathing problems. Water, juice and chicken soup are tasty remedies.
- Get lots of rest! This will help your body channel all it's energy into helping you get better and killing the flu virus.
- Antiviral medicines (such as TamiFlu) can be used, but antibiotics are useless against influenza and should not be taken. They are only helpful after the acute phase is over and bacterial complications have become present.
- Wash your hands frequently, to keep them bacteria free and keep from spreading the virus to others.

Prevention

The best way to avoid getting the flu virus is to receive the proper treatment if you are a high risk person, or if you are around high risk people. Getting a flu shot each year before flu season will give you a 70-90% chance of not contracting the virus. This should be done before flu season as it takes adults about 2 weeks to form the antibodies after receiving the vaccine. The shots are administered from mid-October to mid-November. It is also important to note that you CANNOT contract influenza from the flu shot. Soreness at the injection site or a slight fever for a day or so may occur in young children who have not been exposed to it before, but these are only side effects. It is also good to note that you should not receive a vaccination shot if:

- You are severely allergic to eggs, as the flu viruses are grown in hens' eggs. These reactions are rare.
- You are in the first trimester of your pregnancy, unless your doctor advises you otherwise.

If you cannot receive a vaccination there are drugs that can protect against a disease, these are known as antivirals. If you have questions about these you should talk to your doctor before flu season begins. If you have received a vaccination, after flu season has begun and you are at high risk of becoming infected with the virus (chronic illness, age 50+, young children, etc.) then you should look into taking these drugs until your body has made the antibodies and has had time to build up a defense against the virus.

Chapter 36

Insect and Snake Bites

Why are they Dangerous?

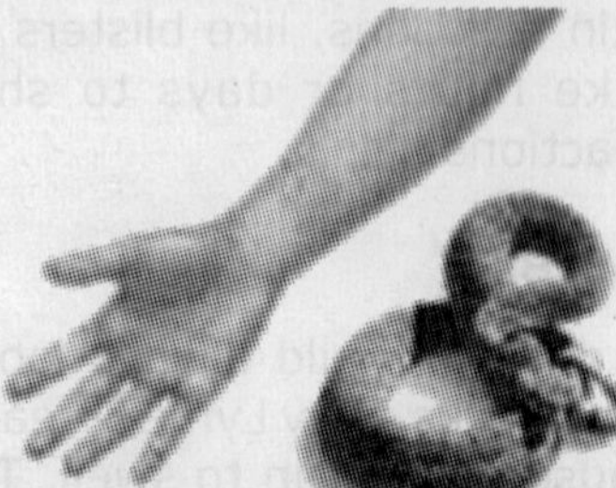

Insect bites and stings carry the risk of allergic reactions, infections and skin injury. The bites introduce a venom to the body that will often cause the skin around the bite to swell and itch. When bites are received wash the area with water and soap, then apply antibacterial cream and a bandage. Below are directions for caring for more specific types of bites.

For information of **Human and Animal** bites go to **bites**.

Insect Bites

1. If the reaction is mild, apply a paste made from baking soda and water, wet cloth or ice (in a bag or cloth to avoid cold injuries).
2. If **allergic** reaction seems to be taking place seek medical help as soon as possible, severe reactions should get help immediately.
3. Seek medical help if bite becomes infected, or looks like it might.

Spider Bites

1. Keep the bitten area still and hanging down.
2. Apply ice (in a bag or cloth. Do not apply directly to skin).
3. Seek medical attention to ensure spider is not poisonous.
4. If shock occurs take the necessary medical steps.

Bites from Black Widow or Brown Recluse spiders may cause nausea, fever, pain and local skin reactions, like blisters. Spider bites may take hours or days to show any of these reactions.

Tick Bite

A doctor should always look at tick bites, as many ticks carry Lyme Disease, a disease which causes the brain to swell. These bites usually leave a circular skin bump behind.

Because there are several different kinds of ticks, and different diseases they can transmit, we have developed a page dedicated to this topic.

Snake Bites

When you receive a snake bite, your body is introduced to, at times, a powerful venom. It is very important to get immediate medical attention if *any* of the following symptoms occur:

1. Hives
2. Swelling lips, tongue, throat and or eyes
3. Slurred speech
4. Coughing, difficulty breathing, wheezing
5. Numbness and cramping
6. Nausea and vomiting
7. Anxiety, confusion, or unconsciousness.

If you can, try to identify the snake, or take note of it's appearance. This will help doctors determine if the snake is poisonous. If you can't find it, don't bother looking for it. Don't give the person anything to eat or drink, especially alcoholic beverages. If you think the snake was poisonous then you may apply a 'light' tourniquet 2-4 inches above and below the bite area.

Most snakes are not poisonous, and poisonous snakes are not found in Maine or Alaska, but you should still have these bites inspected so you can prevent the spread of bacteria and infection. Getting medical attention quickly is important because the anti-venom serums are ineffective if they are not administered within 12 hours.

Bee Stings

If someone is stung by a bee, the first step is to remove the stinger if it is still present in the skin (this only occurs with the honeybee, who dies shortly after stinging). This should be done by using tweezers, or, if no tweezers are available, scrape it out with a fingernail, or card. It is important never to squeeze a stinger when removing it, as more venom will be injected into the bite. Then wash the bite area with an antibacterial soap then you may apply an antibacterial cream if you want. After the area has been washed, apply ice wrapped in a cloth or in a bag to the skin (do not apply ice directly as it may freeze the skin and cause more damage), the ice will help minimize the pain and swelling.

If you are not allergic to bee stings, you may experience anything from a mild irritation and itching to the swelling of the entire part of the body that was stung.

If you're allergic to bee stings, you could be subject to a very serious (although rare) allergic reaction known as Anaphylactic shock. This reaction can be life threatening and should be taken very seriously. All cases of anaphylactic shock and suspected shock should report to the emergency room as soon as possible. Most allergic reactions to bee stings are not this serious, and vary from person to person, although many people allergic to stings tend to have worse allergic reactions each time they are stung.

How Do You Treat Serious Reactions (Anaphylactic and Non-anaphylactic)?

If you know you're allergic to bee stings, it's wise to carry the self-injectable antidote epinephrine, better known as adrenalin. These prescription kits are sold under the names Ana-Kit, EpiPen, and EpiPen Jr. (for children), among others. These syringes are injected into the front of the thigh, or a muscle and work to constrict the blood vessels before more damage can be done. Most of the kits come with only one syringe and on occasion more than one dose is needed. Because bee stings can happen at almost any time during the spring, summer, and early fall it is important to keep several kits on hand, especially if medical help is out of reach, for example camping trips, hikes, and on vacations where territory and bugs are unfamiliar. Keep kits at home and in the car, and if your child is allergic, leave a kit with the school nurse. Although this drug may stop a reaction and make you seem alright it is very important to go to your doctor anyway as soon as possible to be sure. In some cases the epinephrine is not enough and intravenous fluids or other treatments are needed. ALL cases of anaphylactic shock, or suspected cases should report to the emergency room **immediately!** The longer you wait the more damaging the effects.

If you or someone you know or live with is at risk of going into anaphylactic shock it is important to know how to use the syringes. Ask your doctor for information about classes you can attend to learn how, when, and where to administer these shots and save a life. It is also advised that a Medic Alert bracelet or necklace be worn.

Signs of Anaphylactic Shock

Reactions of this kind usually occur seconds or minutes after the sting is received, although a few cases have not reacted for up to 12 hours. When one goes into anaphylactic shock, the blood vessels dilate and begin to leak into the surrounding tissues, which may affect some organs. Below are signs and symptoms to look for:

- The skin is the first place to look. Hives, itching, swelling, redness and a stinging or burning sensation may appear. On the flip side, skin may also appear extremely pale.
- Because the blood vessels are leaking a person may feel lightheaded or faint. Some people will lose consciousness because of a rapid drop in blood pressure.
- Sometimes the throat, nose, and mouth become swollen and breathing passages become obstructed. The first signs of this are usually hoarseness or a lump in the throat. In some cases the swelling is so bad the air supply is cut off and the person experiences severe respiratory distress.
- Another respiratory problem could be the constricting of the airways, giving someone the chess tightness, wheezing and shortness of breath commonly associated with asthma.
- People may experience cramping (in women pelvic cramps may develop), diarrhea and nausea and vomiting.
- Especially if the allergen was swallowed, the gastrointestinal tract often reacts.
- Sweating.
- Rapid pulse.

Causes of Anaphylactic Shock

It is important to note that this allergic reaction (which, again, is very rare), is not caused only by bee stings. This reaction can be sparked by an injection, inhaling, swallowing, and being exposed to an allergen that the person is known to be allergic to. Injected allergens could be bee stings, as mentioned, certain vaccines prepared on an egg medium, penicillin, dyes used in diagnostic x-rays, and allergen extracts used in the diagnosis and treatment of allergic conditions. They can also be sparked by food allergies, even if only a small bite is taken. Skin contact with foods rarely causes an anaphylactic reaction. Foods that are commonly associated with this reaction are peanuts and nuts, seafood, and in children particularly, eggs and cows milk. Inhaled anaphylactic reactions are rare, but have occurred from the inhalation of particles from rubber and latex gloves.

Prevention of Anaphylactic Shock

The most important part of prevention is avoiding the allergen as best as you can. For food allergies and insect bites this may be particularly difficult as food is presented in many different ways, and insects are all around you. For some people immunotherapy is key. This therapy introduces small amounts of the allergen to the person and increases the dose over time. This is a lengthy treatment and takes at least five years, however it can be an invaluable form of protection as it is almost 100% effective.

If your allergy involves bee stings it is important to note a few things about the bees. Honeybees can only sting you once, their stingers get stuck in the skin and they must tear away that part of their abdomen to escape. The bee dies shortly after delivering the sting. Luckily honeybees are not aggressive, like some of their relatives, wasps, hornets, and yellow jackets tend to be, these bees will only sting if they are disturbed or injured. The most common sting from these bees is when they are stepped on. The best way to avoid that is to keep shoes on while walking or playing in areas where honeybees forage, such as clover patches and flowerbeds.

Another few things to note about bees (and other stinging insects), is that they are attracted to bright colors and strong scents. Insects seeking nectar are drawn towards bright colors, and perfumes. If you are allergic to these stings it is recommended that you avoid hairspray, perfumes, and colognes and, in the case of bees, bug spray. Bug spray will not deter bees, and since the scent is strong they may even be attracted. You should also avoid areas where food is open to the environment such as garbage cans, dumps, picnic areas etc. Another interesting fact about bees and color, is that black is an irritant to bees, while blue is a comforting color, it is important to remember this when selecting bathing attire.

Chapter 37

Knee Pain

Definition Knee pain

Knee pain refers to any aching or burning pain in the knee joint. Knee pain can be a symptom of numerous conditions and diseases, including knee stress, osteoarthritis, injury, gout, infection, and bursitis.

Description

Knee pain is very common. Each year, millions of people visit the doctor for knee pain. It is the most frequent reason for visits to an orthopedist (bone and joint surgeon).

To understand the various causes of knee pain, it is important to know how the knee functions. The knee refers to the joint where the femur (thigh bone) meets the tibia (largest lower leg bone). In front of this joint lies the patella (knee cap). The joint is lined by a membrane called a synovial sac. The synovial sac produces synovial fluid which acts as a lubricant much in the way that oil lubricates the moving parts of machinery. Other tissues that make up the knee joint include cartilage, muscles, tendons, and ligaments. The upper end of the tibia has cartilaginous shock absorbers called menisci (singular meniscus). Other protective structures are the bursae, which cushion areas of friction in the joint. Most of the muscles involved with joint mobility originate in the thigh, cross the knee joint, and attach to the tibia.

The knee supports two to three times a person's body weight. It is a complex joint that allows for a considerable range in mobility. In addition to simple flexion (bending) and extension (straightening) movements, the knee joint is designed to allow for rotation, gliding, and rolling movements. To allow for complex mobility and joint stability, joint strength is sacrificed, making the knee vulnerable to injury.

Causes & symptoms

Knee pain is a symptom of many different diseases and conditions. Short-term knee pain may be the result of excess stress on the knee. Possible causes of knee pain include:

Arthritis: Osteoarthritis (joint degeneration), rheumatoid arthritis (joint inflammation), and septic arthritis (joint infection) can cause knee pain.

Bursitis: Inflammation of the bursae of the knee can cause knee pain. Bursitis, sometimes called house-maid's knee, can be caused by infection, gout, rheumatoid arthritis, injury, illness, or chronic irritation (crawling or kneeling).

Cysts: A cyst is a fluid-filled sac. Cysts associated with the knee can cause swelling and knee pain or discomfort.

Fracture: Breakage or crack in any of the bones associated with the knee joint can cause knee pain.

Gout: A faulty chemical process leads to high levels of uric acid in the blood which causes inflammatory arthritis, crystal deposits in joints, joint destruction, and joint pain.

Ligament injury or instability: The ligaments supporting the knee may be injured or strained by persons who participate in sports, particularly football, rugby, lacrosse, basketball, skiing, soccer, and volleyball. Other accidents can also cause ligament damage.

Loose bodies: This condition refers to any loose objects that float around the knee and cause problems. They also are called "joint mice" because of their elusive nature.

Meniscus conditions: Damage, usually in the form of a tear, to the menisci can result from degenerative changes associated with advancing age or sports-related injury. Sports that commonly cause menisci damage include football, basketball, soccer, tennis, lacrosse, and skiing.

Osteonecrosis: Degeneration of the bones associated with the knee cause pain and deformity.

Patellofemoral pain. Also known as anterior knee pain syndrome, this condition is characterized by pain around the knee cap. The exact cause of patellofemoral pain is unknown but is probably related to muscle inadequacy, lack of flexibility, rapid growth, or bone positioning.

Diagnosis

Knee pain can be diagnosed and treated by an orthopedic surgeon. Diagnosis is based primarily on medical history and physical exam. The diagnosis begins with a detailed medical history to fully characterize the knee pain. The knee will be bent to determine the range of motion and palpated (felt with the hands) to detect the presence of any abnormalities. The physical exam may include any of a number of different tests designed to detect injuries by manipulating the knee and leg. X rays may be taken. In some cases more advanced testing may be carried out using magnetic resonance imaging (MRI), computed tomography (CT), or contrast arthrography (x ray following injection of a contrast solution).

Treatment

Most alternative treatments for knee pain aim at reducing pain, inflammation, and stiffness. Persons experiencing long-term or severe knee pain should consult a physician to determine the underlying cause.

Herbals

Several herbal remedies are recommended to relieve knee pain. Some remedies are used externally, while others involve internal use of herbs.

Various other alternative treatments that can be helpful in relieving knee pain include:

Acupressure: Pressing the Stomach 36 point located below the knee caps tones muscles and relieves joint pain anywhere in the body. Pressing the Spleen 9 points located below the kneecap on the inside of each leg relieves knee pain.

Acupuncture: Inflammation and pain may be relieved by acupuncture. The large intestine meridian is the most effective channel for pain relief. A National Institutes of Health consensus panel found that acupuncture may be an effective treatment for osteoarthritis pain.

Aromatherapy: Aromatherapy with essential oils is sometimes recommended. The essential oil of peppermint relieves pain and decreases inflammation: The essential oil of rosemary relieves pain and relaxes muscles.

Exercise: Regular moderate exercise can reduce pain by improving the strength, tone, and flexibility of muscles. The endorphins released while exercising may also be helpful.

Food therapy: Following a detoxification diet may restore nutritional balance to the body and relieve joint pain: Animal proteins may induce joint pain caused by such inflammatory conditions as arthritis, so following a vegetarian diet may be helpful.

Homeopathy: Rhus toxicodendron is recommended for joint and arthritis pain that is worse in the morning and relieved by warmth. Kali bichromium is indicated for persistent, severe pain. Other homeopathic remedies can be designed for specific cases by a homeopathic practitioner.

Hydrotherapy: A warm compress can relieve joint stiffness and dull pain. A cold compress or ice pack can relieve sharp, intense pain.

Magnetic therapy. Magnetic fields may increase blood flow and block pain signals.

Massage: Joint pain may be relieved by massaging the area above and below the painful joint. Massaging with ice packs may interfere with pain signals and replace them with temperature signals.

Reflexology: Knee pain may be relieved by working the knee reflex points.

Rolfing: This deep, sometimes painful, massage therapy may speed healing and reduce pain.

Supplements: Knee pain may be relieved by taking vitamin C to promote healing, the B vitamins to balance the nervous system, which reduces pain, and calcium to increase bone strength.

Allopathic treatment

Knee pain may be relieved by taking such nonsteroidal anti-inflammatory drugs as acetaminophen (Tylenol), ibuprofen (Advil, Motrin), or naproxen (Aleve). More severe pain may be treated with such prescription pain relievers as tramadol or a narcotic. Additional treatment for knee pain depends upon the underlying cause and may include injection of drugs into the knee, surgery, wearing a brace, and/or physical therapy. Surgical treatment depends on the cause; but in the case of osteoarthritis, some patients face actual replacement of the joint. However, in 2002, a new device was introduced that postponed the need to replace an arthritic knee. The device is made of chrome and fits between the natural structures of the knee.

Prevention

Strengthening the leg muscles may help prevent knee pain caused by overworking the joint. In addition, a stronger knee may prevent injury to the joint. Squats are an easy exercise that will strengthen the quadriceps (front thigh muscles) and hamstrings (back thigh muscles). The yoga warrior posture strengthens the muscles around the knee and increases range of motion.

Chapter 38

Labor Pain and Delivery

Delivery of a healthy newborn is a much-awaited event in every family at the end of pregnancy when labor sets in. Pregnancy being a natural or physiological process every person tends to expect a favorable outcome hoping for a "normal" (vaginal) delivery in every case. This is true in nearly 80% of all pregnancies which reach term and result in the delivery of a healthy baby from a healthy mother.

However the onset of labor is usually spontaneous and unpredictable, occurring at any time of the day or night. Labor is also a very dynamic process subject to many variables such as the power (uterine contractions), passage (maternal tissues especially bony pelvis) and passenger (baby/fetus). There should be adequate preparation to handle the situation once labor sets in and delivery is anticipated because there is a wide range of locations where labor and delivery are managed in our country ranging from home to the best equipped hospital.

One should know that NORMAL DELIVERY is a retrospective diagnosis and these words are used only when a healthy mother delivers a healthy baby and neither of them suffers any complications, hence this outcome cannot be predicted accurately before or during the process of labor. Let us understand a few basics about labor before we read about providing first aid during labor.

How to know the onset of Labor?

The exact cause for onset of labor is unknown though a number of theories are suggested, hence it is difficult to accurately predict the time of onset of labor.

Complaints of mother (Symptoms)

1. Painful, intermittent, regular tightening of the abdomen (uterus) which may be accompanied by pain starting in the lower back and radiating towards the front and going down to the thighs.
2. Mucoid vaginal discharge may be passed, at times accompanied by blood ("show")
3. If leakage of clear watery fluid occurs, it suggests that the bag of waters (membranes) has ruptured which may occur with or without pains and this should definitely not be ignored in the absence of pains.

Examination findings (Signs)

1. On feeling the mother's abdomen, uterus can be felt to contract for some time and then relax before the next contraction. Such contractions occur at regular intervals and during this time the mother also complains of painful sensation. From abdominal palpation, a trained or experienced person can also get information about the presentation (head or other part above pelvis), position of the baby, and amount of fluid (liquor) around the baby, heart rate of baby and how much the baby has entered the mother's pelvis from above.
2. Internal examination is possible only by an experienced / trained person who can gain information about condition of cervix (i.e. mouth of uterus), its dilatation, shortening, softness, presence of membranes, presentation of baby (head or some other part like buttocks, feet, hand), station of presenting part / position of baby, pelvic adequacy.

After complete examination, it is usually possible to estimate an expected time of delivery anticipating that labor is expected to progress normally.

Certain High-risk situations

- Early leaking (PROM/EROM)
- Excessive Bleeding before delivery (APH) / after delivery (PPH)
- Abnormal Presentation of baby (Malpresentation such as Breech, Transverse Lie, Cord Prolapse, Hand Prolapse) see Figure 1.
- Maternal Convulsions
- Prolonged Labor (more than 18 hours in Primigravida, more than 12 hours in Multigravida)
- Maternal shock (e.g PPH, Uterine Inversion)
- Retained placenta
- High risk pregnancy such as Twins, Previous Cesarean Section, Medical Disorder such as Cardiac disease, Diabetes Mellitus, Hypertension, RH negative mother, IUGR, Premature Baby.

Preliminary requirement in first aid for laboring women

- Arrangement for transport.
- Accompanying relative or attendant.
- Paramedical / medical personal during transfer from peripheral health care facility to higher centre.
- Availability of emergency drugs, intravenous fluids etc.
- Arranging donor for blood transfusion if patient is bleeding or looks pale.

Principles of providing 5 cleans during labor

Delivery kits prepared and kept ready containing a clean sheet, fresh razor blade, gloves, clean linen, thread for tying the cord.

1. CLEAN SURFACE
2. CLEAN HANDS
3. CLEAN CUT
4. CLEAN CORD
5. CLEAN TIE

Stages of labor

First stage: starts from beginning of pain which causes dilatation or opening up of mouth of uterus (cervix) and ends at full dilatation of cervix.

Second stage: starts at full dilatation of cervix and ends at delivery of baby.

Third stage: starts after delivery of baby up to expulsion of placenta.

Fourth stage: Observation for around 2 hours after delivery especially to see for bleeding and watch mother's pulse, blood pressure and start breast feeding of baby.

First aid at home/outside a hospital

The ideal place for delivery would be a fully equipped medical institution. However many women in our country especially in rural population either do not have easy access to health services or their relatives prefer delivery at home. In such cases services of dais or TBAs (Traditional Birth Attendants) who may be trained or untrained, are usually sought for. An experienced TBA can usually judge which women are not suitable for home delivery and they can advice timely transfer to a medical institution.

- A laboring woman requires privacy and isolation to maintain her dignity.
- Principles of asepsis and antisepsis must be strictly maintained during examination and delivery.
- Preparation of clean surface and other material during conduction of delivery must be kept ready.
- The laboring lady should be encouraged to

have frequent and adequate fluid intake and light diet to supply energy and avoid dehydration.

- An experienced and sympathetic companion can offer psychological support and provide back massage during pains.
- If an experienced and trained person is available for monitoring the progress of labor they should watch for any early signs of developing complications and advise timely referral where necessary.

First aid in hospital

History taking: Complete history is asked to know duration of pregnancy from date of LMP, time passed since onset of pains/ leaking/ bleeding. History of Tetanus Toxoid immunization status, any specific complaints such as swelling of feet/ hands, dimness of vision, headache, breathlessness, fever. Any preexisting medical disorder such as thyroid, diabetes mellitus, hypertension, Valvular heart disease, renal disorder, previous obstetric history such as total no. of pregnancies, living children, mode of earlier deliveries

Examination: General examination to note presence of anemia, edema, lymphadenopathy, peripheral signs of cardiac failure, dehydration. Vital signs such as temperature, pulse, blood pressure, respiratory rate. Systemic examination includes abdominal examination:- size of uterus, presentation, position of baby, liquor amount, contractions-frequency, intensity, duration, heart sound of fetus (FHS) and its rate vaginal examination:-to know stage of labor (I or II), presenting part, position, presence of membrane, station of presenting part, adequacy of pelvis. Documentation of all above in notes accompanied by date and time of examination to evaluate further progress, Partogram (graphic representation of labor) to be plotted if possible.

I.V line with 18 Guaze IV cannula may be secured especially in high risk cases such as grand multipara, twins, hypertensive, previous cesarean section, malpresentation, antibiotic administration is needed in cases of prom / erom, anemia. Cardiac disorder, diabetes mellitus that are at risk of infection. If hemoglobin and blood group are not documented preferable to do so at the time of admission, allow ambulation and fluid intake and light diet only in low risk cases in early stage of labor. Maintain strict asepsis and antisepsis especially during every vaginal examination which should be preferably 4 hrs apart unless indicated at earlier time.

When IInd stage starts cervix is fully dilated and mother feels the need to bear down and push the baby out voluntarily along with every contraction. Baby descend in to pelvis and head can be seen at outlet of vagina at which time person attending delivery should assist the mother and prevent uncontrolled delivery of the baby which may cause tears over her private parts.

In III stage watch for separation of placenta and then help in expulsion when seen at vaginal outlet. Never apply too much pull to extract placenta if it is not coming out easily otherwise uterus will get inverted out vagina and heavy bleeding can start with patient going in to shock.

Immediate care of baby/ newborn: remove secretions from mouth and nose, should cry immediately after birth, keep in warmth, wipe completely starting from head and remove wet cloth from body after wiping, tie cord 5 inch away from naval/ umbilicus and cut extra length with clean, fresh blade. Start breast feeding as soon as mother is comfortable.

Few problems encountered during labor and after delivery

1. Diagnosing labor
2. Calculating expected time of delivery

3. CPD (Cephalo-pelvic disproportion-mismatch between large size of baby in relation to maternal pelvis)
4. Abnormal progress of labor
5. Fetal distress
6. Cord/Hand prolapse
7. Managing twin delivery
8. Patient requiring Cesarean section
9. Tears and trauma to passage/maternal tissues
10. Baby resuscitation
11. PPH
12. Infection after delivery

Conclusion: Labor is a natural yet unpredictable process and till the outcome is a healthy mother with a healthy baby, it cannot be accurately predicted that every delivery will be a 'normal delivery'. From onset of pains up to delivery of baby and then the placenta, labor is a very dynamic series of events. Hence basic knowledge is helpful when faced with an emergency situation away from a hospital to know what first aid to provide to the laboring women so that she may reach a hospital in time and safe or she can be assisted to have an uneventful delivery under less than ideal or favorable circumstances such as are available in a hospital.

Food in Pregnancy

A Woman's healthy pregnancy is dependent on what she eats every day. Hence a healthy diet should be followed when she is pregnant. The diet that she follows during her pregnancy not only enhances her health. It plays a vital role in the baby's health too. The following four basic food groups should be included in your diet strictly.

Starch Filled Food: Vegetables should be your first preference when you are pregnant. Starch filled foods like potatoes, rice, chapatis, oatmeal etc should be made as an important part of your daily diet. As these suggested foods are rich in many calories and vitamins it's advised to strictly have them.

Dairy Foods: Although dairy products are important in your diet, it's advised to take low-fat products. Products like milk, yogurt or cheese are rich source of calcium, which are very essential for your bone. Also these dairy products have other essential minerals like zinc, iodine and magnesium, which are very much needed for the babies' health.

Fruits and Vegetables: Eating lots of fruits and vegetables will not only provide you with minerals and vitamins. It will also give you fiber that helps in good digestion. Hence will prevent constipation.

Meat, Fish and Alternatives: Eggs, meat, fish, nuts, pulses, peas etc are very rich in nutrients. These foods along with your dairy and starch filled foods give the baby a healthy building block. These foods are good source of iron, zinc, vitamin A and B.

Although these are the certain foods that you should follow during your pregnancy, it is also important to avoid certain foods. The food list that you should avoid during pregnancy includes:

1. Strictly avoid having sweet and sugary foods like biscuits, cookies, cakes or chocolates. Although sugar contains calories, it does not have nutrients that your body need.

2. Avoid liver and liver products, although liver products are rich in Vitamin - A, it can ruin your baby's health.

3. Avoid fatty foods like chips, pastry, chocolates etc. Although fat rich foods are high in calories too much can ruin your health. It can lead to heart diseases and excess weight gain.

Chapter 39

Lice

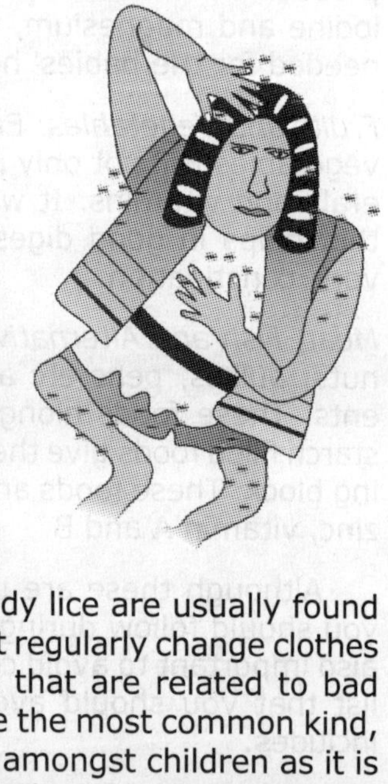

Lice are a common annoyance found most often amongst school children. These parasites live by infesting humans and sucking their blood. There are three types of lice—head, body, and pubic. Pubic lice, or crabs, are found in the pubic hair regions and are spread through close personal contact as well as sexual contact. Body lice are usually found on persons who do not regularly change clothes and are the only lice that are related to bad hygiene. Head lice are the most common kind, and are very popular amongst children as it is easy for them to jump from head to head and spread rapidly throughout schools. As soon as lice are discovered they should be treated to avoid further spreading of the parasite. If your child has lice you should notify your school officials as soon as possible to make sure that it hasn't begun to spread.

What to Look For

- *Head lice:* Intense itching on the scalp, especially behind the ears and at the nape of the neck. Head lice are pretty easy to see, they're roughly the size of a sesame seed and are white. Their seeds are smaller and harder to see.

- *Body lice:* Unexplained scratch marks on the body, hives, eczema, and red pimples.
- *Pubic lice:* Continual itching around the pubic area.

Treatment

To treat head lice, you can go to your pharmacy to get some good over the counter treatments. These treatments are usually shampoos, which will kill the existing lice and any eggs. In the meantime, it is advisable that people infected with lice stay away from others to avoid spreading the lice. Continually wash and sterilize all bed linen, clothing and towels and face washers.

To treat body lice, wash the entire body with soap and water. If this is not effective, you may have to use an insecticide preparation, which usually kills all the lice. As above, wash all clothing and bed linen, towels and face washers.

Pubic lice are treatable by over-the-counter preparations and the same applies as above. Also you should let any partners know about the lice so they can take all the necessary treatments and precautions.

See A Doctor If

Scratching has led to infection or the lice will not go away.

Chapter 40

Lightning

What To Do Around Lightning...

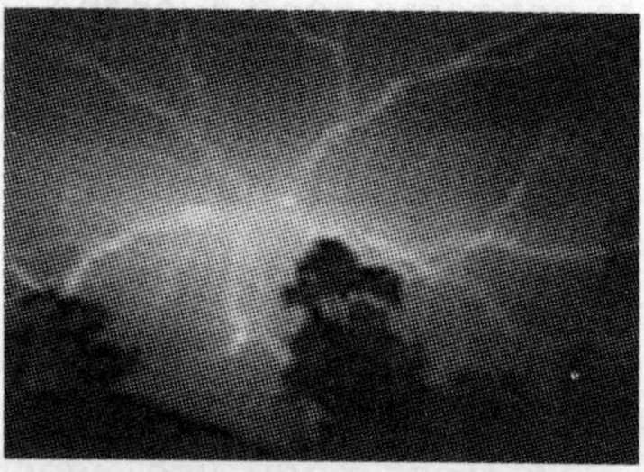

All thunderstorms produce lightning and, in India large number iof people are killed and hundreds more are injured each year. To avoid getting struck, take the following precautions:

- Understand that if you hear thunder, you risk being struck by lightning if you are outdoors. Lightning can strike as far as 10 miles from any rainfall or storm clouds.
- Keep an eye on the sky when participating in outdoor activities, or planning them. Also make sure to listen to the weather forecast before you go out.
- Do not resume activities until at least 30 minutes since the last thunder or lightning was seen or heard.
- If you hear thunder or see lightning get to a safe place at once. The safest places are inside a sturdy building. But if you don't have one around...
  - —A hard topped metal vehicle is ok, just be sure to keep the windows closed and not to touch any of the metal in the car.
  - —If you're in the woods, stand under a cluster of smaller trees that are close together and assume the following posi-

tion. Crouch down on the balls of your feet, put your hands on your knees and bend your head down. Make yourself the smallest target possible and minimize your contact with the ground. NEVER lie flat on the ground, no matter where you are.
  - If you're in a place where there are hills and ravines, move into a ravine and assume the position above.
  - If you are in a field assume the position above.
- Stay away from things like:
  - Tall isolated trees.
  - Small shacks/sheds/unstable buildings.
  - Towers/utility poles.
  - Stages.
  - Boats, pools, and anything else in or very close to open water.
  - Small metal vehicles like scooters, bikes, motorcycles, and golf carts.
  - Anything metal like bleachers, fences, rails, scaffolding, pipes etc, lightning/electricity can travel a long way through metal.
  - Clotheslines are also good transmitters of electricity.
  - Golf courses, golf clubs, carts, metal golf cleats etc. Every year golfers are killed and injured because they do not get off the courses in time.
  - Other people. If you are in a group spread out several yards away from each other.
- If you feel your hair stand on end, beware! You may be about to be struck by lighting.

What To Do if Someone is Struck?

A lightning strike has a different effect on the body than an electric shock and therefore is treated differently. Unlike electric shock, lightning has less effect on the internal nerves and muscles and the people struck carry no electrical charge, which means that they are safe to touch. Similar to electrical shock, the person may be mildly or severely burned. Strike victims need immediate attention and aid, and those that appear "dead" can often be revived and should be attended to first. Quickly (but not too roughly) shake all victims lying on the ground, if they respond in any way move on to the next victim. If people are breathing on their own they will probably be ok, so lay them on their side in the recovery position. Even if they are unconscious they should be alright. You also want to move the victims to a safer place, as the storm is still a threat as lightning CAN strike the same place twice.

Lightning fatalities are usually due to cardiac arrest, or a heart attack. By performing **CPR,** or rescue breathing, depending on whether you can find a pulse or not. If you have several victims at hand, attend to those without a pulse first. If you are not the only person giving aid, or the victims are breathing on their own, call doctor as soon as possible. If you have several victims not breathing, or without a pulse, move them close together and go between the two, giving CPR to both of them. The people who are not breathing should recover quickly and be able to breath on their own after a few minutes of rescue breathing.

It is also good to know that the lightning bolt does not have to hit you to kill you. If the ground is wet, the electricity will travel out a short distance in waves that can affect those standing on the ground. People can be killed by this and are to be treated the same as if they had been directly struck by lightning.

Although most lightning strike victims recover, many are left with disabilities, which is why it is so important to heed the warning signs of an oncoming storm.

Chapter 41

Medicine Safety

Understanding how your medicines work, and being alert to the following things can save your life, and help avoid medicinal mishaps. Medicine safety is no joke, read below for tips to keep you safe and informed.

When You're Still in the Doctor's Office

Questions to Ask Your Doctor and Other Tips...

- Ask your doctor for the medicine that offers the best balance of price and results or outcomes. This tells your doctor in a clear way that treatment goals need to be set, evaluated, communicated and achieved.
- If you're older (over 60) or have kidney disease be certain to ask if the new medications being prescribed will be removed by the kidneys. If this will happen your doctor will most likely want to adjust the dosage.
- Be sure to discuss with your doctor how often you'll need to take the medication. Be honest, if you don't think you'll remember three times a day perhaps there's another medicine for the same problem you'll only need to take once a day. You should 'always' take your medicine as directed on the bottle.
- Ask for the name of the disease the medicine treats to be put on the label. This way if you're taking several medicines you won't risk getting them confused. It will also give the pharmacist an extra check when it comes to filling prescriptions and making sure they're giving you the correct drugs.

- You may wish to ask about side effects, if a certain drug will make you dizzy or tired and you need to take it in the mornings before work, you way want to try a different drug that will allow you to function properly. Some drugs have side effects that are worse than the thing they've been prescribed to cure, so knowing this may make you decide to use a different drug.
- It's also important to find out how soon you can expect to see results and what you should do if the medication doesn't seem to be working.
- While talking with your doctor, show him that you're really interested in your health, and making sure you understand what he or she is telling you. take notes, repeat directions and other information, and ask questions-even if you think they may seem foolish or trivial. Feel free to also inquire as to whether they have any printed information on your medicines on hand. It shows your doctor you care and keeps you safe and informed. To make sure you don't forget something you may want to bring a list of questions with you before you visit the doctors office.

When You Go to the Pharmacy

- When your pharmacist hands you your prescription bag it's often stapled shut- open it up before you walk away. Inside it is your prescription and a brief patient info sheet. Your pharmacist can give you lots of information, and answer your questions about your medications. So if you have any questions about the medication, interactions, or other directions your doctor might have failed to mention, take this opportunity to ask them.
- Read the label when you look at your prescription. It seems simple, but many people don't do it. Reading the label will give you very valuable information—such as taking the

medicine with food, and not taking it along with other medications. Ask if you should avoid certain foods, beverages, other medicines, or activities while you are taking the drug. Question anything you don't understand or that doesn't seem right. Be especially alert to unexpected changes, such as receiving a prescription refill that seems to have a different strength or appearance from your original prescription. If you have questions don't hesitate—Ask.

- Use the same pharmacy for all your medicines. Again this seems simple, but again it's something overlooked by many people. Using different pharmacies means that when having prescriptions filled for new drugs a single pharmacy might not have a list off all the medications you're currently taking. This makes it easy for mistakes to happen. You could be prescribed a medicine by one pharmacy that will interact with one you're already taking that comes from a different pharmacy. Medicine reactions can be very dangerous, so use one pharmacy for all your medicine needs to keep yourself safe. It also gives you an opportunity to develop an good relationship with your pharmacist, they'll be familiar with your medicines which will further decrease the risk of error.
- Another way to avoid interactions is by having your medications mapped. This shows all the drugs you're taking, prescription, non-prescription and herbal, lists side effects, interaction notices, and maps out a logical daily routine for taking your medicine. All of this is on a single sheet of paper as opposed to the multiple pieces of paper that you get for individual prescriptions that you need to organize yourself. This is a fast and simple way to keep you safe and give your doctor and pharmacist and extra final check.
- If a medicine you're on is life sustaining, or you're deathly allergic to a certain type of

medicine, you may want to invest in a medicine alert bracelet, tag, or card. These can be worn or kept in a wallet and if anything happens to you they'll let the medical response teams know what they need to do to help you.

When you Get Home

- Organize your medicines, if you've had them mapped then you've got a handy daily schedule telling you when you need to take your medicine. makes several copies of this in case one gets lost. If you keep a profile of the drugs you take be sure to keep it updated. Make a list of everything you're taking- prescription, non-prescription, herbal, medicinal foods, etc. and share it with your doctor and pharmacist this will help prevent drug interactions.
- Learn the names, doses, and strength, of the drugs you take.
- Take your medications exactly as your doctor and the label on the bottle prescribe. Doing this ensures that the medicine will work the way it's supposed to, and keeps you safe from bad interactions and other complications. Don't take to little, as it lessens the effect of the medicine, and don't take too much as it could be toxic. Occasionally missing a pill is also big deal—some medicines really do need to be taken every day. talk to your doctor to find out about how your medicines will react if missed. Also make sure that you finish a prescription you've been given unless instructed otherwise. If you're unsure if you were supposed to finish it or not call your doctor.
- If you realize you have more questions once you get home, don't hesitate to call your doctor or pharmacist. It is also important to call them before adding any other drugs (even non-prescription and herbal) to your daily drug regiment. If you're doctor or pharmacist won't make time to answer your

questions you may want to consider finding some new health care providers who will make time for your questions—which are important.

Reactions

- If you think you may have had a reaction, no matter how minor—a headache which was not in the listed side effects, a sudden appearance of a rash, etc. call your doctor immediately to set up an appointment. If the reaction seems moderate to severe call doctor or have a friend drive you to the nearest ER. Even if it turns out to be a false alarm, always be aware of things like that. Also, when you go to the doctor don't just tell them about the new medicine you've been taking, give them a list of everything so that they can check for drug interactions. If you've had a reaction your medications need to be changed, so don't hesitate. Minor reactions will get steadily worse and lead to bigger problems.
- If you are older and on medications, be careful. Some medications can make the elderly and those with a weak immune system miserable. The side effects of many drugs will leave these people bedridden, sick, and generally unhappy. the elderly especially are at risk because as you age your body adapts and reacts differently to medications. So if 6 years ago you took a medicine that worked for you very well, and you start taking it again, now as a senior citizen, you may see and feel considerably different. In situations like this you may not think to ask your doctor many questions about the drug because you've taken it before. But it's important to understand that while the drug hasn't changed your body has, and the two will interact differently and the medicine needs to be reevaluated to make sure it is the correct medication for your current state and situation.

Travelling Safely with Medications

- **Many medications can cause "photo-sensitivity", or increased sensitivity to sunlight.** Even if you don't usually **sunburn**, taking medications that cause this reaction could greatly increase your chances of getting a bad burn. Your pharmacist can advise you about whether your medication can cause photosensitivity and recommend the right SPF (skin protection factor) for your skin type.
- **If you are flying, keep your medications in your carry-on luggage so that you have access to them during your flight and will not lose them in the event that your luggage gets lost.** Plus, keeping your medications with you helps prevent exposure to extreme temperatures in the baggage compartment, which can alter the drug's effectiveness. Keep in mind that airport security requires that your medications be transported in their original, labeled containers.
- **If your medication requires you to use a syringe-insulin, for instance-you may need to carry your prescription with you to ensure that you can pass through airport security.** The American Diabetes Association recommends that people with diabetes be prepared to provide airport security personnel with copies of prescriptions for diabetes medications and supplies as well as complete contact information for the doctor who prescribes the insulin.
- **Make sure that you carry your doctor's and your pharmacy's phone numbers with you when you are away from home.** In case you lose your medications, you may need a new prescription. You should also keep on hand a list of all your prescriptions.
- **If you are traveling through several time zones, consult with your doctor or pharmacist to work out a specific plan for adjusting the timing and dosage of your**

medications. This will prevent you from taking too much or too little.

- **If you are visiting a foreign country, beware of buying "over-the-counter" medications**. Many medicines that are available by prescription in the United States are available "over the counter" in other countries. Some of these medications could have different ingredients, and may not undergo comparable quality control. Buying these medications could put you at risk for allergic reactions, drug interactions, or other problems.
- **If you are visiting a hot, humid climate, be sure to keep your medications in a cool, dry place out of direct sunlight**. Never store medications in the glove compartment of your car. Also, because of the heat and humidity that build up in a bathroom, it is the worst place to store medication whether you are at home or on the road.
  - Take along more medication than the number of days you've planned to be away. This will allow you to be prepared for unexpected delays.
  - Joint and muscle aches
  - Seizures
  - Drowsiness
  - Stiff neck and joints
  - Dislike of light
  - Fever
  - Septicemia.

And in Young Children

- High pitched moaning or whimpering
- Dislike of being handled
- Fidgety and fretful
- Very tired, weak, drowsy even when awake
- Blank starring expression
- Arching back, and neck retraction
- Fever with possibly cold hands and feet
- Refusing food or vomiting

- Pale blotchy skin
- Septicemia.

Septicemia is blood poisoning. This can develop very quickly and is marked by red blotchy rashes all over the body. As soon as a single rash is seen rush to the emergency room, or call for medical aid! These rashes will stay red (rather than turn white) when pressed upon. A simple test is to take a drinking glass and press it against the rash to see if it changes color. **This rash is a sign of bacterial meningitis**.

Treatment

Leave treatment of meningitis up to the professionals. If you suspect a case of meningitis get the person to the doctor sooner rather than later. That can make all the difference! Meningitis can happen to anyone anywhere, and bacterial meningitis cases are most often found on college campuses among freshmen.

Recovery

Recovery from bacterial meningitis is often a long, slow and painful process both physically and mentally for those involved. Meningitis can leave people with irreversible brain damage and loss of hearing among many other things.

Muscle Cramps

Muscle cramps are common discomforts that everyone has had to deal with at one time or another. Here are some signs of a muscle cramp:

- A sharp, sudden, painful spasm, or tightening of a muscle, (especially common in the legs).
- Muscle hardness.
- Twitching of the muscle.
- Persistent cramping pains in lower abdominal muscles.
- Sometimes occurring when a muscle contracts with great intensity and stays contracted, refusing to stretch out again.

Causes

Imbalances in certain minerals, body fluids, hormones, and chemicals which allow the lengthening and contracting of our muscles to occur can prompt spasms and cramps. As well as this, malfunctions in the nervous system itself can also cause problems. Excessive physical activity and hormonal imbalances causes us to sweat, which brings about the loss of many essential minerals (such as potassium) our muscles need.

Traditional Treatment

- For everyday muscle cramps, there really isn't any medication specifically for them. Try to stretch the muscle and massage out the cramp it you can.
- Muscle cramps can also be caused by a lack of potassium and vitamin E, so eating something like bananas or pineapple can help to replenish the minerals you've lost. Calcium is also thought to help prevent muscle cramps, so drink your milk!
- If you take vitamin E supplements it will help prevent nighttime muscle cramps, which can be quite an annoyance.

Prevention

- Drink 6 to 8 cups of water every day.
- Be sure to get enough potassium, vitamin E, and calcium into your system.
- Be sure to warm up before exercising.

When to Seek further Professional Advice

- If you suffer from frequent or severe cramps, see your doctor. And severe cramps in your chest, shoulders, or arms can be symptoms of a heart attack; call immediately for medical help.
- Your muscle cramp lasts more than an hour.
- Your cramp is in your chest or arms.

Chapter 42

Meningitis

What is Meningitis/Classification

Meningitis, some forms of which are known as the "college killer", can be a life threatening illness if treated incorrectly. First, what is it? Basically it is an inflammation of the delicate membranes (the meninges) that cover the brain. There are several kinds of meningitis, viral and bacterial.

Viral meningitis is more common, and is rarely fatal. If treated properly the person will make a full recovery. It is spread like the flu, by coughing, sneezing, or exchanging germs in other ways. Antibiotics cannot defeat the virus, but a vaccine may be available. Ask your doctor if you have questions.

Bacterial meningitis is less common, but is very dangerous and can be fatal. This form of meningitis is caused by a bacteria and is spread much the same way as viral meningitis. It cannot live outside the body for long, and cannot be picked up from water sources. Bacterial meningitis can kill in as little as 24 hours, or take as long as two days to become potentially fatal, so time is incredibly valuable if this illness is suspected. Irreversible brain damage can be caused in as little as couple hours in more severe cases. Antibiotics can be used to treat this virus, but no vaccine is currently available.

Symptoms

In both cases the symptoms are flu-like, and may not appear all at once. (Non flu-like symptoms below are marked with an *. These symptoms may be signs of bacterial meningitis.)

- Coughing
- Sneezing
- Vomiting
- Headache
- Joint and muscle aches
- Seizures*
- Drowsiness
- Stiff neck and joints
- Dislike of light*
- Fever
- Septicemia*.

And in Young Children

- High pitched moaning or whimpering*
- Dislike of being handled*
- Fidgety and fretful*
- Very tired, weak, drowsy even when awake
- Blank starring expression*
- Arching back and neck retraction*
- Fever with possibly cold hands and feet
- Refusing food or vomiting
- Pale blotchy skin*
- Septicemia*.

Septicemia is blood poisoning. This can develop very quickly and is marked by red blotchy rashes all over the body. As soon as a single rash is seen rush to the emergency room, or call for medical aid! These rashes will stay red (rather than turn white) when pressed upon. A simple test is to take a drinking glass and press it against the rash to see if it changes color. **This rash is a sign of bacterial meningitis**.

Treatment

Leave treatment of meningitis up to the professionals. If you suspect a case of meningitis get the person to the doctor sooner rather than later. That can make all the difference! Meningitis can happen to anyone anywhere, and bacterial meningitis cases are most often found on college campuses among freshmen.

Recovery

Recovery from bacterial meningitis is often a long, slow and painful process both physically and mentally for those involved. Meningitis can leave people with irreversible brain damage and loss of hearing among many other things.

Chapter 43

Migraine

Migraines are the worst most painful sort of headaches. These headaches are fierce and severe and can last for several hours or a couple days. Migraines are caused by the constricting and swelling of blood vessels on one side of the brain, and it is thought that they may be genetic, this, however, is still uncertain.

Signs and Symptoms

Migraines are often preceded by:
- Feelings of **nausea** and sickness
- Blurred vision
- Flashing lights in front of the eyes.

Once they have begun, migraines...

- Start as a sharp throbbing pain on one side of the head which may spread as the headache worsens.
- The person may become very nauseas which may lead to vomiting.
- The person may be very sensitive to light, noise, and certain foods.

Treatment

There are many different treatments available by prescription from your doctor. Usually these medications are prescribed when the migraines are very severe or you suffer 2 or more each month. Another thing you can do to help ease the pain is gently massage your face with your fingertips. Do this by gently massaging your temples in a circular motion; repeat in the hollows at the sides of your eyes (by your nose), behind your ears, and over your neck.

People suffering from migraines have identified the following foods and other things which have been found to trigger migraines.

- Foods with caffeine (coffee, soda, chocolate)
- Citrus fruit
- Aged cheese
- Processed meat
- MSG (food additive)
- Red wine
- Foods with high levels of magnesium
- Missing meals
- Stuffy rooms
- Dry wind
- Changes in season or altitude
- Birth-control pills or other hormonal changes
- They may also occur after intense emotional periods, such as anger or excitement.

Chapter 44

Muscle Cramps

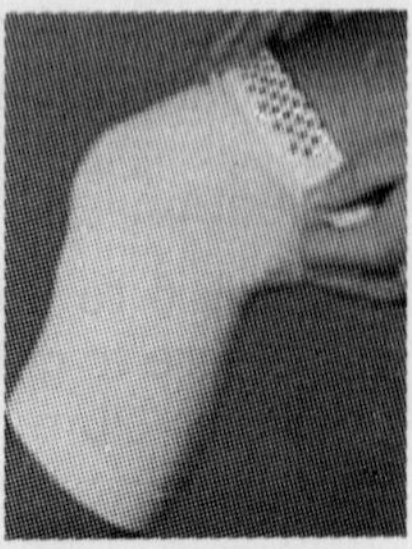

Muscle cramps are common discomforts that everyone has had to deal with at one time or another. Here are some signs of a muscle cramp:

- A sharp, sudden, painful spasm, or tightening of a muscle, (especially common in the legs).
- Muscle hardness
- Twitching of the muscle.
- Persistent cramping pains in lower abdominal muscles.
- Sometimes occurring when a muscle contracts with great intensity and stays contracted, refusing to stretch out again.

Causes

Imbalances in certain minerals, body fluids, hormones, and chemicals which allow the lengthening and contracting of our muscles to occur can prompt spasms and cramps. As well as this, malfunctions in the nervous system itself can also cause problems. Excessive physical activity and hormonal imbalances causes us to sweat, which brings about the loss of many essential minerals (such as potassium) our muscles need.

Traditional Treatment

- For everyday muscle cramps, there really isn't any medication specifically for them.

Try to stretch the muscle and massage out the cramp it you can.

- Muscle cramps can also be caused by a lack of potassium and vitamin E, so eating something like bananas or pineapple can help to replenish the minerals you've lost. Calcium is also thought to help prevent muscle cramps, so drink your milk!
- If you take vitamin E supplements it will help prevent nighttime muscle cramps, which can be quite an annoyance.

Prevention

- Drink 6 to 8 cups of water every day.
- Be sure to get enough potassium, vitamin E, and calcium into your system.
- Be sure to warm up before exercising.

When to Seek Further Professional Advice

- If you suffer from frequent or severe cramps, see your doctor. And severe cramps in your chest, shoulders, or arms can be symptoms of a heart attack; call immediately for medical help.
- Your muscle cramp lasts more than an hour.
- Your cramp is in your chest or arms.

Chapter 45

Nausea and Vomiting

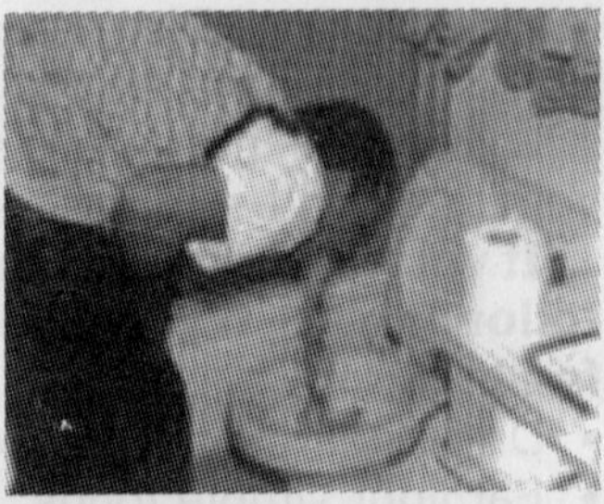

Old or young, when you feel sick, there are few things worse than feeling nauseous and vomiting. Nausea itself is an uneasiness of the stomach, which may or may not lead to vomiting. And although they may feel it, they are symptoms of diseases rather than diseases themselves. They are usually a result of things like:

- Viral and bacterial infections like **colds** and **flu's.**
- Food poisoning.
- Over eating and **indigestion.**
- Certain smells and odors.
- Intense pain.
- High **fever.**
- Emotional stress (like fear or excitement).
- Motion sickness, seasickness, and dizziness.
- Early pregnancy ("morning sickness").
- Cancer treatments like chemotherapy and radiation.
- Exposure to toxins (poisons, chemicals).
- Blocked intestine (rather uncommon, and usually found in early infancy).
- Appendicitis.
- Head injuries, like **concussions**, migraines, brain injury.
- And sometimes they're a sign of more serious injuries like kidney and liver disorders, heart

attacks, brain tumors, gall bladder disease, nervous system disorders, and some kinds of cancer.

Often, if you aren't sure of the cause you can determine it merely from the time when the feelings first occur. If it occurs right after a meal, indigestion, an ulcer, or a mental disorder (such as bulimia) could be to blame. One to eight hours after a meal could indicate food poisoning. Diseases like salmonella may take several days before any nausea is felt.

Luckily, in many cases both nausea and vomiting can be controlled to some degree.

If you're feeling nauseous you can do the following to try and control or stop the feelings:

- Drink clear or cold drinks.
- Eat light simple foods, like saltine crackers, which don't have a strong taste or odor. Take care to avoid sweet, greasy, and fried foods as they will only make you feel worse. Also do not mix hot and cold foods.
- Eat slowly, and have small frequent meals throughout the day as opposed to three larger meals.
- Drink beverages slowly and take small sips, try to drink between meals instead of during them.
- Do not brush your teeth right after eating.
- Avoid activities immediately after eating, instead rest after eating with your head elevated about twelve inches above your feet. Activity may increase nausea.
- If you feel nauseous when you wake up in the morning, have some crackers (like saltines) before getting up and moving about, or have a snack before bed that's high in protein (like cheese, or some lean slices of meat).

If you already feel nauseous and want to avoid the unpleasantness of vomiting, try these tips:

- Drink small amounts of sweet clear cool liquids, like ginger ale, fruit juice (try to avoid citrus—orange, grapefruit—drinks as they are too acidic), etc. Sweet liquids are good for calming the stomach.

- Eating cool sweet things like popsicles may also help to calm your stomach. However do not eat or drink too many sweet things, only have a little at a time or the condition may worsen.
- You can also get some prescription and non-prescription drugs to help control vomiting and nausea related to pregnancy, vertigo, and motion sickness, but make sure you speak with your doctor before starting on any new medication—even if it is over the counter. Also, if you're vomiting due to treatment of another kind (such as chemotherapy) your doctor may be able to prescribe something to control the nausea.

If You Do Get Sick

In most cases vomiting is harmless, but sometimes it can indicate or even cause problems. With vomiting you should always be on the lookout for signs of dehydration, especially with children. Children need to be watched extra carefully because unlike adults, they can't easily recognize the signs and symptoms of **dehydration**. Here are a few of the symptoms to look out for.

- Dry lips or mouth.
- Increased thirst.
- Decreased urination, or urine that is dark in color.
- Sunken eyes.
- Rapid breathing or pulse (mainly in infants).

If diarrhea occurs along with the vomiting, make sure to keep a very close watch on the person and give them small amounts of clear, cool, sweet drinks. Drinks with electrolytes (like a watered down sports drink).

Consult Your Doctor If

- Vomiting goes on for longer than one day (or if they are very young and it continues for a few hours).
- There is blood in the vomit.
- If the vomiting is occurring because of a known injury, like head trauma or infection.
- The child has not urinated in at 6 hours.
- The person acts confused, lazy or lethargic, and is less alert than usual.
- They have a fever of over 102 Fahrenheit.
- Vomiting and diarrhea are present.
- Severe abdominal pain is present.
- Severe headache or stiff neck is present.
- Feelings of nausea last for longer than one week.

With these exceptions, vomiting can be treated at home. Give the person small amounts of clear liquids, increasing the amount as feelings of nausea subside. This will discourage dehydration. Avoid solid foods until feelings of nausea have totally passed. Also discontinue taking any oral medications, as they may further upset the stomach, but make sure you check with your doctor before doing this.

Chapter 46

Near Drowning

Almost drowning, or near drowning, is a frightening and potentially fatal thing, there are two kinds of this:

"Wet"—Where the person has taken water into their lungs, and the lungs function has been affected.

"Dry"—Less common condition where the airways closed due to spasms induced by water.

When rescuing someone who has nearly drowned, make sure to watch out for your own safety as well, do not attempt a rescue that is beyond your abilities. Let other people help out as well, for example, if you are not physically strong do not attempt to remove someone larger than you from the water, let someone else do this while you wait onshore ready to begin resuscitation.

Symptoms

- Pale cool skin.
- Weak or absent pulse.
- Labored or absent breathing.
- Slightly conscious or unconscious.
- Cyanosis (bluish discoloration of the skin).

Treatment

- Asses the situation quickly, check vitals and if necessary begin **CPR.**
- If needed treat for **Hypothermia.**
- If needed treat for **Shock.**

- If any neck or spinal injuries are suspected try not to move the person unless absolutely necessary. And call for an ambulance.
- When they have begun breathing correctly and are not at risk of shock or hypothermia place them in the recovery position.

It is important to know that near drowning has a large affect of the respiratory system, and if the lungs have fluid in them it may lead to at best pneumonia and at worst a fatal condition known as "late drowning". If someone has suffered from near drowning they should go see as doctor as soon as possible.

Chapter 47

Nosebleeds

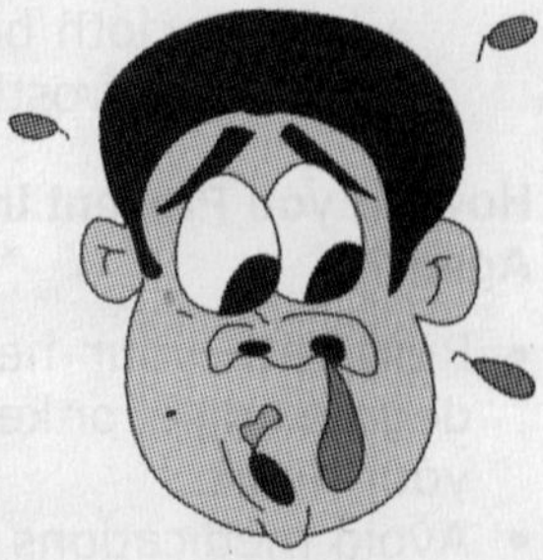

Nosebleeds are a common injury amongst people young and old. The nose is a part of the face rich in blood vessels and any trauma to the face can start a nosebleed. Nosebleeds are also common in dry climates and during the winter months when people are going from the cold to the dry heat of their homes. During these months the nose membranes become cracked and dry. This drying out of the membranes is what causes nosebleeds. People who are taking medications that prevent normal blood clotting are at a higher risk of getting a nosebleed. For these people only a light trauma could spark a nosebleed. Other factors that promote nosebleeds are alcohol abuse, infection, use of blood thinning medications, hypertension, allergic and non-allergic rhinitis, and less commonly, from inherited bleeding problems and tumors.

Stopping the Common Nosebleed

In most cases the common nosebleed is fairly easy to stop, and no medical help is needed.

1. Using a clean cloth, tissue or sterile gauze, pinch the nose together at the nostrils and firmly apply pressure towards the face. Hold like this for at least 8 minutes, or until the nose stops bleeding.

2. Have the person lean forward slightly or sit up straight. Do not let the person lean back, or blood may flow into the windpipe. Keep the head above the heart, or in other words, don't let the person lie down. If they must lie down try to keep their head elevated at a 45 degree angle.
3. Apply crushed ice in a bag or cloth to nose and cheeks. Make sure the ice is in a bag or cloth because direct application may cause frostbite to skin.

How do you Prevent the Nose from Bleeding Again?

- Rest with your head elevated at a 30-45 degree angle, or keep your head higher than your heart.
- Avoid medications which will thin the blood (such as aspirin), but make sure to contact your doctor before stopping taking any prescribed medications.
- Do not smoke.
- Try not to sneeze. If you must sneeze open your mouth to allow the air another way to escape to avoid upsetting the nose.
- Try not to strain. Heavy lifting/pulling/pushing should be avoided!
- Try to keep to a "cool diet" for 24 hours. Avoid hot liquids.
- Your doctor may recommend a lubricant for the inside of your nose if you are prone to recurrent nosebleeds. This is easily applied with a Q-tip or the tip of a finger. Make sure to coat the middle part of the nose especially, as it is the most vulnerable.
- If it does start up again attempt to clear the nose of clots by sniffing in forcefully. Nasal decongestant sprays may also be used, but if they are used for an extended period of time they may become addictive.
- And if all else fails repeat the above steps for stopping common nosebleeds.

When to go to the Doctor?

If bleeding keeps occurring and you feel faint or weak from blood loss then you should report to your doctor, or local emergency room. There they may stop the bleeding with a heating instrument and blood tests may be taken to check for disorders. If bleeding still persists then the doctor may place nasal packs, which compress the blood vessels and stop the bleeding. And in rare situations surgery is needed to plug the nose and stop the bleeding.

What are these nasal packs? What happens if I get them?

If your doctor has placed these packs within your nose you will need to return to the hospital in 2-5 days to have them removed. Nasal packs are made of a spongy material that compress the blood vessels and are usually only used when more conservative methods fail. When you go for your removal appointment make sure you have arranged rides to and from the hospital as you will be prescribed pain medications and antibiotics as needed. It is also advised that you continue to avoid blood-thinning medications unless otherwise noted by your doctor.

When these packs are placed, it isn't uncommon for the nose to drain some blood-tinged material. This can be caught by taping a folded piece of gauze under the nose like a mustache. In some cases your doctor will permit you to clean your nostrils with hydrogen peroxide soaked Q-tips.

Chapter 48

Poison

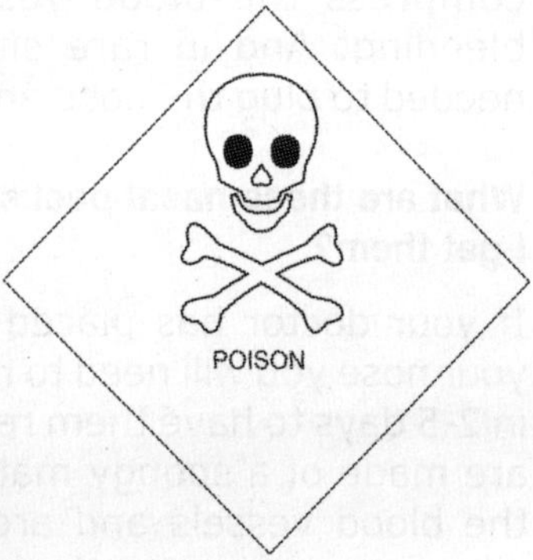

We live in a world where we are surrounded by poisons we can inhale them, swallow or ingest them, absorb them through our skin, or have them injected into our bodies. Each year about 2.5 million poisonings are reported to poison control centers and approximately 1,000 of them become fatal. Knowing the signs and symptoms or poisonings, being aware of the poisons in your home, and keeping the number of the poison control center handy. Preventing the poisoning to begin with is the best first aid you can possibly give. Here are some good tips to remember about poisons:

- Just because a package doesn't have a warning label, you shouldn't assume that it's not a poison or that it's safe.
- Symptoms of poisoning can happen instantly or take hours, days, months or even years to become apparent. So if you suspect poisoning for any reason, get help. As the cliché goes—it is always better to be safe than sorry.
- Suspect a poisoning if someone suddenly appears to take ill, or if a person is found

unconscious or 'ill' near a fire, furnace, a car, or in an area that is very badly ventilated

Common Poisons Include

- Medications, one of the reasons you're never supposed to take somebody else's medication because their dosage may not be right for you and can cause serious problems. Medications also need to be stored in safe places so that children cannot access them.
- Household cleaning products and detergents
- Plant/garden products (weed killer, some fertilizers).
- Insecticides, rodent and snail poisons.
- Paints, paint thinners, and lead paint chips (swallowing paint, or inhaling fumes).
- Chemicals found at ones job, or in ones home for use in things like pools (chlorine, rat poison, kerosene etc.).
- Illegal drugs.
- Poisonous plants such as poison ivy—which will cause a reaction, and others which will be toxic if eaten such as some varieties of mushroom or berries.
- Animals with venomous stings, poisonous sprays, bites etc.
- Food that has gone bad, or been cooked incorrectly.
- Carbon Monoxide gas fumes, or other noxious fumes such as those expelled by cars, chemical reactions, or in a fire.
- Some cosmetics can be poisonous if used incorrectly (swallowed/misted in eyes perfumes or aftershaves).

Symptoms

Symptoms of poisoning again may appear instantaneously or the poisoning may be cumulative and symptoms may take years to become apparent. Below is a list of some symptoms that are along the "occur soon after the poisoning" variety:

- Chest pain
- Abdominal pain
- Cough
- Diarrhea
- Confusion
- Bluish lips (cyanosis)
- Dizziness
- Double vision
- Difficulty breathing
- Shortness of breath
- Drowsiness
- Unconciousness
- Weakness
- Headache
- Seizures
- Nausea and vomiting
- Loss of appetite
- Loss of bladder control
- Burns around lips or mouth
- Burning pain in throat or mouth
- Skin rashes or burns
- Stupor
- Irritability
- Muscle twitching
- Numbness or tingling
- Fever
- Pale, cool or clammy skin
- Heart palpitations (a rapid, weak or erratic pulse)
- Unusual breath odor
- Ringing in the ears
- Smell of fumes or odors.

Treatment

A brief list of Do Nots

- Do Not give a poison victim (conscious or not) anything by mouth unless instructed to do so by the poison control center.
- Do Not induce vomiting unless instructed by the PCC. If the poison burned on the way down it could also burn on the way up.
- Do Not try to neutralize the poison with anything you have heard will help, such as

lemon juice or vinegar unless you are instructed too, they could aggravate the situation further.

- Do not wait for symptoms to develop if you suspect a poisoning. Get help immediately, call your local PCC or if the victim is unconscious or the injury seems serious call doctor before the PCC.
- Do Not go by the instructions on a label when it comes to treating poison, as many labels have our of date instructions.

First Aid for Poisoning by Swallowing or Ingesting

- Unless it is necessary to perform CPR first, call the Poison Control Center, or for very serious reactions call doctor, and then the PCC.
- Check and monitor the victim's airway, breathing and circulation. If the victim becomes unconscious or if necessary for other reasons, begin **CPR**. If there is something lodged in the persons throat Do NOT give CPR until the object has been **removed**.
- Try to make sure that the victim has indeed been poisoned, this may be difficult as it is sometimes difficult to tell, especially if the victim in unconscious or very young. Some signs include chemical-smelling breath, burns around the mouth, difficulty breathing, vomiting, or unusual odors on the victim. If possible, identify the poison.
- Only induce vomiting if the poison control center tells you to do so.
- If the victim vomits, protect the airway. If you must clear the victim's airway, wrap a cloth around your fingers before cleaning out his or her mouth and throat to protect yourself from any poison that may have been left in the mouth or throat. If the victim has vomited a plant part, save the vomit, as it

may allow identification by an expert who can then determine an antidote.

- Reassure the victim and keep him or her comfortable. Position the victim on their left side while getting or awaiting medical help.
- Call the Poison Center for any poison taken by mouth, whether it was swallowed or not. Never induce vomiting unless instructed to do so by the poison center or your doctor. You may be instructed to give the victim sips of water or milk.

  CAUTION: Some out-of-date first aid and health information charts may contain incorrect treatment information. DO NOT give raw eggs, salt, vinegar or citrus fruit juices to induce vomiting or to neutralize the poison. These treatments are not only ineffective, but may be extremely dangerous.
- If possible, have the poisonous substance or its container within reach while you are speaking with the Poison Center.
- If you are instructed to go to a hospital emergency department, take the substance or its container with you.

First Aid for Poisoning by Inhalation

For inhalation poisoning:

- Unless it is necessary to perform CPR first, call the Poison Control Center, or for very serious reactions call doctor, and then the PCC.
- Take several deep breaths of fresh air, then hold your breath as you go in. If it is safe to do so, rescue the victim from the danger of the gas, fumes, or smoke. Hold a wet cloth over your nose and mouth. Open windows and doors to remove the fumes. Understand that in very serious situations—such as a fire—you may not be able to rescue the victim, and the safer choice would be waiting for help to arrive then directing them as best you can.

- Avoid lighting a match as some gases may ignite.
- Once the victim has been removed from danger, check his or her airway, breathing, and circulation. If necessary, perform rescue breathing and **CPR.**
- As necessary, perform first aid for skin **burns**, **eye injuries**, or **seizures**.
- If the victim vomits, protect his or her airway.
- Even if the victim seems perfectly fine, get medical help. Sometimes poison symptoms take a while to surface.
- DO NOT use Ipecac Syrup or activated charcoal in the first aid treatment for poisoning unless advised by the Poisons Control Center.

Poison on the Skin

- Remove any contaminated clothing, taking care to avoid contact with the chemical.
- Flush the skin with cool-lukewarm running water for 20 minutes.
- Call the PCC to find out if any additional aid needs to be given. If the reactions to the poison seem serious, or from a chemical you are unfamiliar with call doctor or go to the ER.
- If possible, have the poisonous substance or its container within reach while you are speaking with the Poison Center.
- If you are instructed to go to a hospital emergency department, take the substance or its container with you.

Poison in the Eye

- Remove contact lenses if worn.
- The eyes must be irrigated for a full 15/20 minutes with cool-lukewarm water.
- Eyes do not have to be held open continuously during the flushing treatment; opening and closing the eyes repeatedly

during irrigation helps carry the water to all parts of the eye.

- Call the PCC to find out if any additional aid needs to be given. If the reactions to the poison seem serious, or from a chemical you are unfamiliar with call doctor or go to the ER.
- If possible, have the poisonous substance or its container within reach while you are speaking with the Poison Center.
- If you are instructed to go to a hospital emergency department, take the substance or its container with you.

Prevention

- Be aware of poisons in and around your home. Take steps to protect young children from toxic substances. Store all medicines, cleaners, cosmetics, and household chemicals out of reach of children, or in cabinets with childproof latches.
- Be familiar with plants in your home, yard, and vicinity. Keep your children informed, too. Remove any noxious plants. Never eat wild plants, mushrooms, roots, or berries unless you know what you're doing.
- Teach children about the dangers of substances that contain poison. Label all poisons.
- Don't store household chemicals in food containers, even if they are labeled. Most non-food substances are poisonous if taken in large doses.
- If you are concerned that industrial poisons might be polluting nearby land or water, report your concerns to the local health department or the state or federal Environmental Protection Agency.
- Store medicines, chemicals and household products safely out of reach and out of sight of children, up high (at least 4½ ft) in a locked or child resistant cupboard.
- Do not take other people's medicines.

- Separate medicines from household products.
- Use medicines and chemicals safely. Be sure that all products are properly labeled and in their original containers.
- Clean out your medicine cupboard periodically. Take out-of-date medicines to a pharmacy for disposal.
- Children tend to mimic adults, so avoid taking medicines in their presence.
- Do not refer to medicines as being sweet, or tasting like candy.
- Use personal protection equipment when spraying or painting. Ensure there is adequate ventilation, with circulating air.
- Remove any contaminated clothing immediately.
- Keep everything in original containers never in cups or soft drink bottles.
- Obtain a history-look for empty bottles, containers, and sometimes suicide notes. If possible, ascertain what poison or medicine has been taken, including how much and when.
- The Poison Center recommends that all homes with young children should have a first aid kit that contains both ipecac syrup and activated charcoal. Never use either substance without first calling the poison center or your doctor. By having both items in the first aid kit, you provide poison control staff and doctors with more ways to help you treat a poisoned person.
- Remember, that the PCC is not just for emergencies—it's a great source of information and the people who work there are trained to answer your questions about poisons and how to prevent and recognize problems before they start.

Chapter 49

Rib Injuries

The ribs are fairly resistant to injury, but sometimes accidents happen. The most common injury is a rib fracture, and these are more commonly found in adults. The reason for this is that children have more elasticity in their bones, which causes them to break less easily. Another common injury to the ribs is muscle strains.

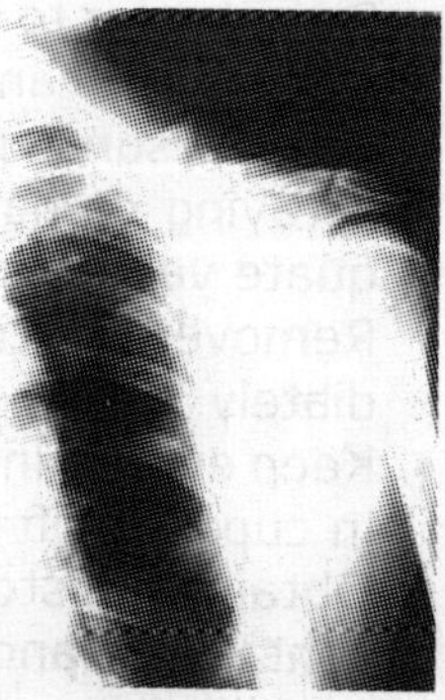

Rib Fractures

Rib Fractures are usually caused by a direct blow (or fall) to the ribs. Ribs 4-9 are the most commonly broken because they would receive the most pressure in the event of a direct blow. The following are symptoms of a broken rib:

- Severe localized pain.
- Sharp pain with any motion of the chest (breathing, coughing, sneezing, laughing).

See your doctor if any of the following things occur, as they may indicate complications from the fracture such as a pierced lung:

- You become short of breath, or your breathing is labored and difficult
- You become lightheaded
- The area swells
- When the injured area (place where the pain is greatest) is gently pressed a "crunching" sound is heard.

- The pain seems very severe or "deep"
- There is pain in your abdomen
- You are coughing up blood
- There is blood in your urine.

Remember, if you are unsure if you have broken a rib you should see a doctor to make sure. Also keep in mind that about 25% of rib fractures will not show up on an x-ray. These injuries cannot be cast, due to their position, but to ease the pain and discomfort a elastic ace bandage may be wrapped around the persons chest. If you are able to continue doing most of your everyday activities with only minimal pain it's a good sign. If there is a deep pain, or you are unable to partake in everyday activities it may be a sign of a worse injury and you should consult your doctor.

Treatment

One of the first things you should do is apply ice to the injured area. Icing the injury early on can help reduce the inflammation and pain. Over the counter pain medication may also be given to ease the pain. If it hurts to breath and move, which is likely, then you should wrap and elastic ace bandage around the persons chest to help restrict movement. Discourage the person from taking deep breaths and partaking in activities (if you are hiking, take a break, and move slowly when you begin again). Encourage the person to take shallow breaths, go slowly, and rest often. Loosen the bandage around their waist once an hour and have them take a couple deep breaths, it may hurt, but it should be done anyway. Apply ice packs (wrapped in a cloth, rather than placed directly on the skin) for about 30 minutes every two hours for two or three days.

As for movement and activities, a simple rule applies: if it hurts, don't do it. The injury should heal in 4-6 weeks depending on the severity of the break. The pain of the injury will gradually decrease.

Muscle Strains

Muscle strains are another common rib injury. The muscles affected in this injury are more often the muscles attached to the rib cage than the muscles along the chest wall. They can be injured by over stretching, or by sudden violent contractions. Sports like tennis, golf, baseball, and basketball can cause this sort of aggravation. Occasionally strains are confused with a heart attack because of the severity and location of the pull.

Chapter 50

Seizures

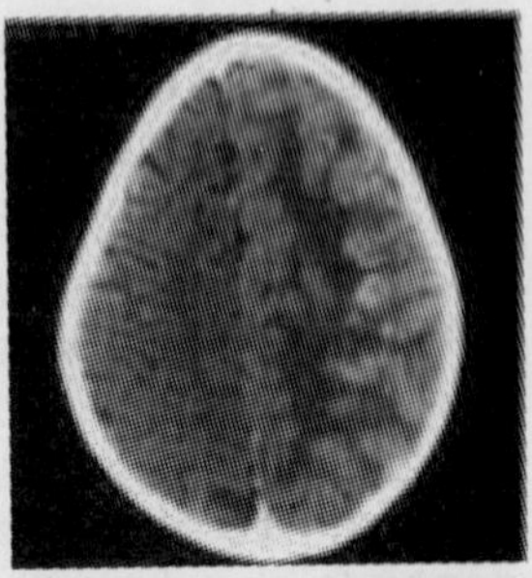

Epilepsy is a chronic neurological condition characterized by recurrent seizures that are caused by abnormal cerebral nerve cell activity. Epilepsy is classified as idiopathic or symptomatic. A nerve cell transmits signals to and from the brain in two ways by (1) altering the concentrations of salts (sodium, potassium, calcium) within the cell and (2) releasing chemicals called neurotransmitters (gamma aminobutyric acid). The change in salt concentration conducts the impulse from one end of the nerve cell to the other. At the end, a neurotransmitter is released, which carries the impulse to the next nerve cell. Neurotransmitters either slow down or stop cell-to-cell communication (called inhibitory neurotransmitters) or stimulate this process (called excitatory neurotransmitters). Normally, nerve transmission in the brain occurs in an orderly way, allowing a smooth flow of electrical activity. Improper concentration of salts within the cell and overactivity of either type of neurotransmitter can disrupt orderly nerve cell transmission and trigger seizure activity.

Certain areas of the brain are more likely than others to be involved in seizure activity.

The motor cortex, which is responsible for body movement, and the temporal lobes, including the hippocampus, which is involved in memory, are particularly sensitive to biochemical changes (e.g., decreased oxygen level, metabolic imbalances, infection) that provoke abnormal brain cell activity.

Seizure Phases

A seizure often has three distinct phases: aura, ictus, and postictal state. The first phase involves alterations in smell, taste, visual perception, hearing, and emotional state. This is known as an **aura**, which is actually a small partial seizure that is often followed by a larger event. The seizure is known as **ictus**. There are two major types of seizure: partial and generalized. What happens to the person during the seizure depends on where in the brain the disruption of neural activity occurs. Following a seizure, the person enters into the **postictal state**. Drowsiness and confusion are commonly experienced during this phase. The postictal state is the period in which the brain recovers from the insult it has experienced.

Types

The International Classification of Epileptic Seizure identifies seizure types by the site of origin in the brain. The two main categories of seizures include partial seizures and generalized seizures. A partial seizure can evolve to a generalized seizure. There are several subtypes of each. Only the most common are described here.

Partial Seizures

The site of origin is a localized or discreet area in one hemisphere of the brain. The two most common types of partial seizure are simple partial and complex partial.

Simple Partial

These produce symptoms associated with the area of abnormal neural activity in the brain: motor signs, sensory symptoms, autonomic signs and symptoms (involuntary activity controlled by autonomic nervous system), and psychic symptoms (altered states of consciousness). There is no impairment of consciousness in simple partial seizures.

Complex Partial

Impairment of consciousness, characteristic of complex partial seizures (CPS), results in the inability to respond to or carry out simple commands or to execute willed movement, and a lack of awareness of one's surroundings and events. Automatisms may occur. An automatism is a more or less coordinated, involuntary motor activity. A simple complex seizure may begin as a simple partial seizure.

Generalized Seizures

At the onset, seizure activity occurs simultaneously in large areas of the brain, often in both hemispheres. Seizures can be convulsive or nonconvulsive. The two most common types are tonic-clonic and absence.

Tonic Clonic (Grand mal)

There is loss of consciousness during the seizure. The tonic phase, consisting of increased muscle tone (rigidity), is followed by the clonic phase, which involves jerking of the extremities. Automomic symptoms may also be present.

Absence (Petit mal)

This type occurs most often in children, usually beginning between the ages of 5 and 12 years and often stopping spontaneously in the teens. The loss of consciousness is so brief that the child usually does not even change position. Most absence seizures last 10 seconds or less.

There is no postictal state, but the person usually lacks awareness of what occurs during the seizure.

Myoclonic

These seizures are so brief that they may go unnoticed. They involve sudden muscle contractions that occur much more rapidly than clonic activity and are often confused with tics. Myoclonic seizures occur at all ages and are associated with epileptic syndromes such as West syndrome and Lennox-Gastaut syndrome.

Syndrome and Situation-Related Epilepsy

Infants and Children

Epilepsy is one of several symptoms that occur in West syndrome and Lennox-Gastaut syndrome. West syndrome, also called infantile spasm, is a rare disorder of infancy and early childhood. It is characterized by epilepsy, hydrocephalus, congenital anomalies, and mental retardation.

Lennox-Gastaut syndrome usually develops between the ages of 1 and 8 years old and is characterized by atonic, absence, and myoclonic seizures. Many of these children are developmentally delayed and have behavioral problems.

Adults

Several medical conditions may precipitate epilepsy in adults, notably withdrawal from chronic alcohol and drug abuse, eclampsia, and stroke.

A Seizure is a miscommunication between the nerve cells and the brain. When a seizure occurs normal brain functions are impaired and sometimes brain damage can occur. There are two kinds of seizures, **General** (tonic-clonic or 'grand-mal') and **Partial** (temporal lobe). General seizures affect small areas of the brain while Partial seizures affect the whole brain. Seizures usually last only a few minutes (in between 1 and 10) and must run their course before they end.

Causes

Seizures can be caused by:

- High fevers (especially in infants and young children) these are known as "fever fits"
- Epilepsy
- Brain injury, strokes
- Infection
- Poison
- Snakebites (or bites from other venomous creatures)
- Shock
- Heat stroke
- Vaccinations
- Reactions or overdoses to medication or drugs
- Diabetes
- Trauma
- Reye's syndrome.

Treatment

Symptoms and treatment are as follows:

General

- The person may yell or cry out
- Stiffen
- Difficulty breathing (look for pale or bluish skin)
- Jerking motions
- Falling
- May last 1-4 minutes.

Treatment

- Remain calm
- Move all sharp edged objects out of the persons way to help keep them from injuring themselves

- Monitor their breathing
- Do not try to restrain the person, you cannot stop the seizure
- Do not force anything into the persons mouth or give them anything to eat or drink.

Once the Seizure has Subsided

- Help the person lay down and place something soft under their head.
- Turn them to one side so they don't risk choking on their saliva.
- Remove tight or restricting clothing and jewelry.
- The person will probably feel confused and disoriented.
- They will also be very tired, let them sleep but stay with them until they have awoken and are fully awake and alert/aware.
- Do not give them anything to eat or drink until they have fully recovered.

Partial

- The person may experience convulsions (violent shaking and seizing, uncontrollable jerks and twitches)
- Glassy stare
- May give no response, or an inappropriate response when questioned
- May sit, stand or walk around aimlessly
- Make lip smacking or chewing noises
- Appear to be drunk, drugged, disorderly, or even psychotic
- Fidgety
- Crying out
- Falling over
- Losing consciousness
- Body may stiffen.

Treatment

- Remain calm, and call doctor (this may not always be necessary in the case of epileptics, but is always necessary if the person is diabetic).

- Move all harmful objects out of the persons way, or try to direct them away from them vocally (if they are not convulsing).
- Do NOT try to restrain the person.
- Observe their behavior, in more severe cases this may become very important information.
- Be very gentle with the person, and do not be too physical with them.

Once the Seizure has Subsided

- The person will be very sleepy, let them sleep
- They may have a headache.
- Give them no food or drink until after they have rested and are fully alert and recovered.
- The person may be confused and disoriented.
- Turn them to one side so they don't risk choking on their saliva.
- Remove tight or restricting clothing and jewelry.

Chapter 51

Shock

What is Shock?

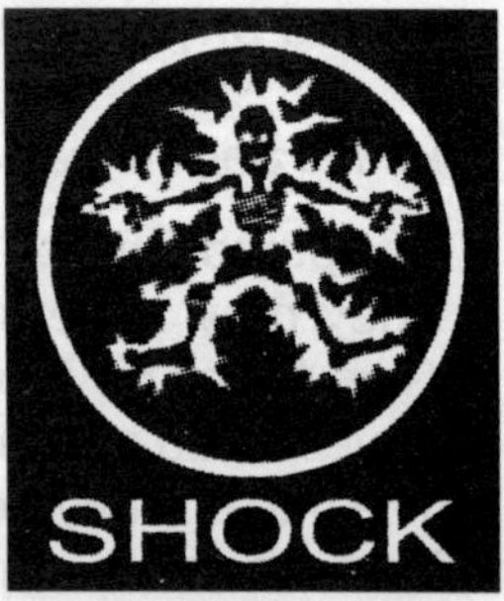

Shock is what happens when the heart and blood vessels are unable to pump enough oxygen-rich blood to the vital organs of the body. Although every illness and involves shock to some degree, it can be a life threatening problem. The best way to protect people from the serious damages that shock can have on the system is to recognize the signs before the person gets into serious trouble. In most cases, only a few of the symptoms will be present, and many do not appear for some time. The most common symptoms are:

- Pale, cold, clammy and moist skin
- Vacant or dull eyes, dilated pupils
- Anxiety, restlessness and fainting
- Weak, rapid, or absent pulse
- Shallow, rapid, and irregular breathing
- Nausea and vomiting
- Excessive thirst
- Person may seem confused or tired
- Loss of blood pressure.

Classification of Shock

Hypovolemic Shock: This form of shock is brought on by a decrease in the amount of blood vessels or other fluids in the body.

Excessive bleeding from internal and external injuries, fluid loss due to diarrhea, burns, dehydration, and severe vomiting usually cause this kind of shock.

Neurogenic Shock: In the case of neurogenic shock, the blood vessels become abnormally enlarged and the pooling of the blood disallows an adequate blood flow to be maintained. Fainting is an example of this sort of shock, as the blood temporarily pools as the person stands. When the person falls the blood rushes back to the head and the problem is solved.

Psychogenic Shock: This shock is more common, and is known as a "shock like condition". It is produced by excessive fear, joy, anger, or grief. "Shell shock" is a psychological adjustment reaction to stressful wartime experiences. Treatment for shell shock is limited to emotional support and help from a medical facility.

Anaphylactic Shock: This form of shock is brought on by an allergic reaction from a food, bee sting or other insect bite, and inhalants. For more information on the care and treatment click the link below.

Treatment of Shock

1. Call doctor (or your local emergency help provider) for help.
2. Lay the victim face up, on a blanket or coat if possible, and raise the feet above the head unless they are fractured. If the person is bleeding from the mouth or vomiting, tilt their head to the side to avoid fluids going into the lungs and airways. If you are unsure of injuries keep the person laying flat.
3. Loosen tight clothing, braces, belts, jewelry etc to avoid constriction of the waist, neck and chest.
4. Keep the victim comfortable and warm enough to be able to maintain their own body heat. If possible, remove wet clothing and place blankets beneath the victim. NEVER

use artificial sources of heat. If they are bleeding severely do not apply heat to the wounded area as it will prevent the blood from clotting as easily.

5. Check for other injuries, such as **bleeding** and **burns** and treat the other injuries according to first aid procedures. If possible try to splint **sprains** or **broken bones**. *If you are unsure of how to do this, leave them as they are to avoid further damage.*
6. If they claim they are thirsty moisten their lips with water but DO NOT give them anything to drink, as it may induce vomiting.
7. Try to keep the victim calm, excitement and excessive handling will worsen their condition try to assure them help is on the way.

Remember, if you can perform these actions before shock has completely developed you may prevent its occurrence and if it had developed you may stop it from becoming fatal. If shock is left unattended to the victim will die, it is extremely important that first aid be performed as soon as possible.

Chapter 52

Skin Closure Strips

What are Skin Closure Strips?

Skin closure strips are a relatively new alternative to stitches. They are used to comfortably secure, close and support small and long cuts and wounds while promoting fast natural healing. The strips themselves hold the lacerated skin firmly together while the breathable bandage creates a moist environment while protecting the wound from dirt, water, and germs. These kinds of sutures also help prevent scarring and risk of infection.

What Types of Wounds are They Used on?

These can be used on small and long cuts that need more support and are deeper or bleeding more profusely than a minor wound. In the case of animal **bites,** deep or puncture **wounds**, serious **burns**, and infected wounds always consult a doctor before applying the skin closure strips. Skin closure strips are not to be used over large areas of the body, or near the eyes. In medical emergencies always consult a doctor first.

How do I Apply and Care for Them?

First stop bleeding and then gently cleanse the wound and surrounding area (about 3 inches in each direction) with water before patting completely dry. For strips and bandage to work the skin needs to be free of oils, creams, and dirt. If you cannot clean out the wound do not use these strips.

Next Apply Strips as Follows:

1. Hold the strips the long way and remove from package.
2. Remove the backing from one end of the strips and firmly place down next to and in the opposite direction of the wound.
3. Line up the skin edges of the cut and, after removing the center piece of backing paper, place firmly (but gently) across the pulled together skin.
4. Once secure remove the last piece of backing and place down on skin on other side of wound.
   The strips should be tight, but comfortable-too tight will only delay healing and cause further damage such as skin shearing and blistering.
5. Next remove bandage from its package and after removing the backing place over the wound in the opposite direction of the strips.
6. Change the bandage covering the strips daily or as needed, but leave the strips as they are. They will remain in place even when the covering bandage is removed.
7. Do not use for longer than one week unless advised by doctor.

If you have even a small worry that the wound could need stitches, or if the wound is bleeding profusely (even after skin closure has been applied), was caused by an animal bite, serious burn, or a puncture consult your doctor as soon as possible. If the wound becomes infected, swells, itches, is abnormally painful, has a burning sensation contact a doctor immediately and discontinue use.

Skin closure strips are also helpful after surgery or after stitches or staples have been removed. They provide extra support for the newly healed skin around the injured area.

Removal

Removing the strips is also easy but should be done with care. Once you reach the wound site be extra careful. Lifting the strips from one end increases the risk of reopening the wound. Instead try holding each end of the strip and removing them at an even slow pace, this will remove some of the stress on the new skin and lower your chances of reopening the wound.

Chapter 53

Sprains and Dislocations

What is Sprain? A Dislocation?

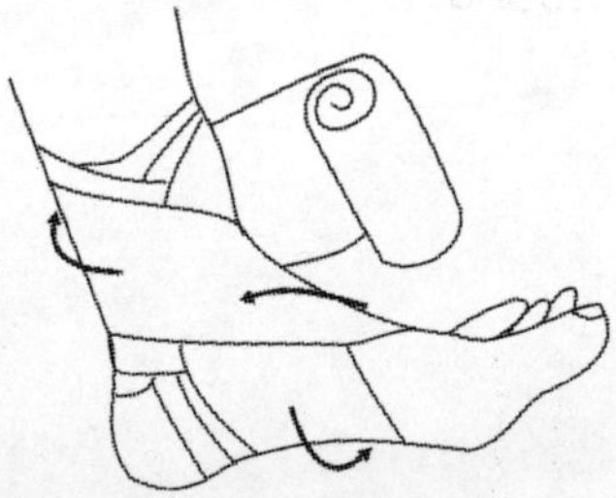

A *Sprain* is an injury to the soft tissue, or ligaments, around a joint. This sometimes happens when someone moves the wrong way and "twists" something.

A *Dislocation* is when the bone becomes separated from the joint it meets, or it pops out of it's socket. This sometimes happens when the bone and joint are overstressed. They an also be caused by contact sports, rheumatoid arthritis, inborn joint defects, and suddenly jerking that arm or hand of a small child. Dislocation is most common in the shoulders, but fingers, hips, ankles, elbows, jaws, and even the spine are also prone to dislocation.

Both of these injuries are commonly confused with fractures (broken bones) because they all exhibit many of the same symptoms.

- Pain
- Swelling
- And an inability to move and bear weight
- A misshapen appearance
- Any discoloration.

Treatments and Warnings

Because of this, the same first aid care can be used for all three of these injuries.

- If you suspect a dislocation do not try to put the bone back into its socket, you may only make the injury worse.
- If you suspect a dislocation in the neck or spine be very careful and do not try to move the person yourself unless absolutely necessary, as damage may have been done to the spinal cord (which may paralyze parts of the body below the injury site.) Also, if you suspect an injury this serious call doctor immediately.
- If the site of injury is bleeding then treat the **wounds and cuts** accordingly, but do not try to reset/reshape the bone or joint. Also look for signs of **shock**.
- If the pulse is weak below the affected area call doctor and loosen all restrictive clothing.
- If the person is in severe pain, or the injury is to the neck, spine, hips, or thigh bone, call doctor.
- If the joint or bone needs to be repositioned, do not give the person anything to eat or drink as it will put off medical treatment.
- Remove any articles of clothing or jewelry covering the affected area, or restricting blood flow to it.
- You may give over the counter pain medications such as acetaminophen and ibuprofen as directed by the doctor. If there is bleeding do not give aspirin because aspirin is a mild blood thinner and will delay clotting.
- Use the PRICE technique:
  - *Protect*—If possible make a splint to help immobilize the affected area. Rulers and cloth, rolled up magazines and a belt, branches and shoelaces; all types of things can be used to make a splint. This will help prevent further damage to the limb. Do not try to reposition the bone/ joint while making the splint.
  - *Rest*—Avoid movement of the injured area and avoid participation in activities where you may be at risk to re-injure yourself

until after the wound had had plenty of time to heal.

— *Ice*—Use ice to minimize swelling. If no ice is available, a bag of frozen veggies is a good substitute.

— *Compression*—An elastic or fabric bandage may help decrease swelling and ease the pain. Ask a doctor before using one and make sure the bandage is not wrapped to tightly, which would hinder circulation.

— *Elevation*—If possible raise the injured limb up above the heart. Support the elevated limb in a sling or under a pillow or folded blanket.

Prevention

- Wear protective gear and padding especially around recently injured areas.
- The Doctor will often tell you how long you should wait before using the injured area again, in a very active way. Take his or her advice as it decreases your chances of re-injury.
- Avoid sports in which you may re-injure the area.

Chapter 54

Suicide

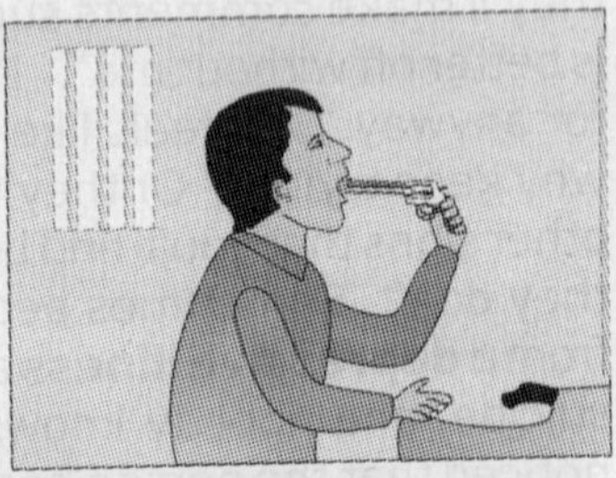

Suicide is a terrifying reality to be faced with-whether you or a friend are contemplating it, or whether somebody you know has attempted it or gone through with it. The subject is unpleasant, and is still considered a taboo subject by the majority of the world. However, its an incredibly important topic that needs to be discussed openly so we can spread the word that help is available, and that you can escape the feelings the depression and suicidal thoughts will you with and return to a happier normal life. It is reported that large number of people in India kill themselves each year (over including teenagers). That seems like a lot, doesn't it? Now triple that number, and you'll be factoring in all the other suicidal deaths that are reported as being accidental each year. It's scary, and downright horrifying—the statistics *and* the fact that despite them, people are still so hesitant to discuss suicide and **depression**—which precedes 95% of suicides. Lets start with some basics, you can find the following on this page:

- An introduction to suicide, things you need to know about it and the people who suffer from it

- Misconceptions about suicide
- The danger signs of suicide
- How you can help, what you can do
- If suicide becomes reality, how to cope, what to say, what to tell children.

One may say, 'If someone I know, like a close friend or family member, is suicidal, I'd know about it. I'd be able to tell', sadly this is sometimes not the case. Sometimes people will drop clues, they'll make comments such as, "Oh, this place is better off without me", "I've got nothing to live for anyway.". "It feels like nothing is changing, why keep trying?" Or they'll exhibit some of the other signs that you'll find below; but sometimes they don't. Sometimes people can be suffering from a **depressive illness** and be contemplating suicide, and nobody knows it. They may have noticed that the person has seemed sad, or less like themselves but they may not realize what is actually going on inside the persons mind because they aren't showing it. Lots of people who suffer from depression try not to show it because they don't want to show weakness or they don't want to upset the people they care about. They may act happy and like nothing is wrong, when in fact they're suffering from a very dangerous condition. Depression is the most misdiagnosed and undiagnosed condition in the US. Depression—untreated or not—can lead to suicide. However, if you do know somebody who may be depressed or feeling suicidal remember—80% of people who die of suicide made some reference about suicide to somebody prior to their deaths. These references should ALWAYS be taken seriously even if they turn out to be false alarms.

People who attempt to commit suicide and fail, what are they trying to say? is it a cry for attention or sympathy? Are they trying to prove something? Yes and no. They aren't necessarily trying to prove anything, but it is a very loud and definite cry for help. It seems obvious, but these attempts should never ever be ignored. Realize that help and aid needs to be given immediately because if they've failed once some people will become more desperate and resort to more dangerous or painful methods to succeed.

Why would someone attempt suicide in the first place? Do they really want to die? The answer here is difficult. Depression is a chemical imbalance and it clouds your mind and changes the way you think. It can also temporarily "shut off" your instinct for survival. Someone who is seriously contemplating suicide is often very depressed, and there is no real way to describe what it feels like. When they reach the point of contemplating suicide—or even self injuries such as cutting or burning—they are in so much pain that it seems like the only way to escape it is by ending their lives, or in the case of cutting, causing an external pain to distract them from the internal pain. People who are contemplating suicide have lost all hope that their lives will ever return to normal and that they will be happy again. Many of them are unable to understand that they can be treated and be 'saved'. *Most people who kill themselves do not want to die, they just want to escape the pain they're feeling*. Most people to not chose suicide, they just give in to the feelings because they do not have the strength to fight them anymore. If they understood that there were other ways out, they would choose life over death.

Why do people who are seeking treatment still try and commit suicide, even if they seem like they're doing better? The road to recovery is a very long one, and there are many ups and downs along the way. Sometimes people who are depressed cannot see any improvement, or just simply cannot deal with their pain any longer; this may cause them to attempt suicide. Sometimes they are so depressed to begin with that they don't have the physical energy to commit suicide, but once the disease starts to lift, they may gain the energy but retain their feelings of hopelessness which may lead to suicide.

If their mind seems like it's made up, is there any way to stop them or change their mind? YES! Never give up on somebody just because they have decided to give up. People who are considering suicide go back and forth between wanting to die and wanting to live, and if suicide occurs it is likely to happen during a lower than usual low. In fact, you helping them see that there are other ways is helping to turn them away from the destructive decision of suicide and showing them that people do care and want them to be safe. If you think someone has made up their mind get them help as soon as possible.

If someone has been exposed to suicide, either of friends or family members, are they more likely to commit suicide themselves? It's true that suicide can run in families, but this is because depression can sometimes be inherited, and this depression- left untreated—can result in suicide. However, if you are healthy, you are not at risk for attempting it. If you are already depressed when the suicide happens, or had gone through depression before there is a chance that you will be at an increased risk. But if you are receiving treatment for your depression, via medications and/or therapy then you should be all right. Also remember that not everyone who is depressed will have suicidal thoughts.

Why don't people talk about suicides? The majority of people still see suicides (and depression) as a taboo topic, and discourage the discussion of it. This is the wrong approach. By talking about suicide and depression you can teach people to recognize the symptoms, and that they can get help and have other options. Talking about it will not put suicidal ideas into people's heads, talking about it will save lives.

Misconceptions About Suicide

These are from the NAMI Advocates:

1. "People who talk about suicide won't really do it."

   NOT TRUE!

   Almost everyone who has committed or attempted suicide has given some clue or warning. No matter how casual or jokingly they may be stated, always take suicide threats seriously.

2. "Anyone who tries to kill themselves must be crazy."

   NOT TRUE!

   Most suicidal people are not psychotic or insane. They must be upset, grief-stricken, depressed, or despairing, but extreme distress and emotional pain are not necessarily signs of mental illness.

3. "If a person is determined to kill him/herself, nothing is going to stop him/her."

   NOT TRUE!

   Even the most severely depressed person has mixed feelings about death, wavering until the very last moment between wanting to live and wanting to die. Most suicidal people do not want death; they want the pain to stop. The impulse to end it all, however overpowering, does not last forever.

4. "People who commit suicide are people who were unwilling to seek help."

   NOT TRUE!

   Studies of suicide victims have shown that more then half had sought medical help within six month before their deaths.

5. "Talking about suicide may give someone the idea."

   NOT TRUE!

   You don't give a suicidal person morbid ideas by talking about suicide. The opposite is true—bringing up the subject of suicide and discussing it openly is one of the most helpful things you can do.

Signs and Symptoms that someone may be contemplating suicide:

- Talking about suicide.
- Joking about suicide.
- Preoccupation with death (reading or writing about it).
- Statements about being helpless, worthless, or hopeless feelings.
- Statements about being reunited with loved ones.
- Loss of interest in things they care about.
- Visiting or calling people they care about.
- Making arrangements; setting affairs in order.
- Giving things away, or returning borrowed items.
- Doing things, "for the last time".
- Symptoms of **depression.**
- Writing letters or notes that refer to death or the "end".
- Suddenly happier or calmer.
- Self-destructive behavior, this includes drug and alcohol abuse, promiscuity, self-injury and mutilation.
- Risk taking behavior, reckless driving, carelessness in dangerous situations etc.
- Having "accidents" that result in injury, also close calls and brushes with death.
- A history of other suicide attempts.
- Obsession with guns or knives.

What You Can Do to Help?

The best thing you can do for the person who is suffering is by taking all their threats seriously and, if need be, by betraying their trust.

Take suicidal comments and hints seriously! As mentioned before, it is critical, especially in cases where depression is involved that you take suicidal, or death related comments or hints very seriously—it's more than likely that the person saying them is trying to send you a message.

Talk about it with your friend. It's very difficult if you have a friend who is suffering from depression, and it's even harder if you're afraid they may be thinking about suicide. You may feel pulled in two directions, you want to ask them if they're thinking about it, but you're afraid that talking about it will give them ideas. Rest assured that it will not. You should never be afraid to talk to someone you care about if you're afraid they may be contemplating suicide. Not everyone who is depressed thinks about suicide, and many who are do not consider it an option so discussing it will not cause them to think otherwise. In fact it has a healing affect on everyone involved because even if your friend is not contemplating it, it lets them know that you cared enough about them to ask what they know is a difficult question—it lets them know that you're there for them. Not sure how to ask? Just try being straightforward. Ask them, "Have you ever felt so upset that you've thought of suicide?". If they say no, leave the subject, but if you're still unsure keep an eye out for clues that they might drop that show signs of suicidal thought. If they say yes, try and get them to agree to get help, or talk with a doctor. It may also be comforting if you offer to go with them so you can both learn how to fight the depressive and suicidal feelings—it will make them feel like they aren't in this alone. Sometimes your friend will say that yes, they have been, but they don't want you to tell anybody about it. Agree not to tell anybody, and realize that this is one promise you are allowed to break and that by breaking it you are being a better friend than if you kept the secret.

Tell somebody. If you think or know your friend has been contemplating suicide you need to tell somebody—such as a responsible adult who will take you seriously and help your friend get help. Never give up, if you tell an adult, teacher, or other friend and they don't take you seriously or are unwilling to act find someone else who will. Please remember that even if they told you not to tell you are being a true friend and doing the right thing by telling. Here's a brief list of people you can go to:

- Parents, guardians, or other family members.
- Teachers.
- School counselor, nurse, or other school official who might be able to help.
- A psychologist, social worker, nurses at a local hospital.
- Religious clergy (such as your priest, or rabbi).
- Other very close friends. A few of the persons closest friend can be an incredibly powerful support and motivation force to get a person who's suicidal or depressed to seek help. It should be noted that the group of informed friends should be kept small; as such feelings are a very personal matter.

Understand their feelings, and offer to help. Realize first, that you can never understand what they feel like unless you've been there yourself, your friend knows this so don't tell them you understand because it will only aggravate them. Realize also that you cannot just talk your friend through depression, but you can change their mind about suicide- this said understand that no matter how hard you try you do not fulfill the need for the help of a professional who can prescribe medicines and other sorts of therapy that you simply cannot. If your friend does wish to talk about things however don't let the fact that you wont be able to solve everything stop you- listen carefully and try not to judge them. If you see behaviors or hear things that concern you, tell somebody. It is very difficult to discuss these things, because you care about your friend and don't want to see them in pain, and also because they are not pleasant topics to discuss, it's easy to not know what to say or how to broach the conversation. Try simple phrases like these, "I can tell you're really upset, and I'd like to help you, do you want to talk about what's wrong?" "I care about you and I know something has been bothering you, let me help". Often people who are depressed or suicidal feel guilty about many things, including feeling depressed and suicidal. In cases where they mention or show signs that they're feeling guilty tell them that, "it's ok, it's not your fault".

Survival instincts and clear thinking. As a final sum up to this section, try to understand that while suicide goes against basic survival instincts for us, the brain of a person who is suicidal is not telling them that because in many cases the mechanism for survival has been shut off. Most people who are suicidal are so depressed that they see suicide as the only way out of the pain they are feeling and do not realize that, with treatment, they could return to the way their lives were before the disease set in. Because they cannot often realize this it is therefore up to the people who care about them to get them help and keep them alive.

When Suicide Becomes a Reality

Surviving a suicide...the grief that follows:

- Know that you can survive. Though you may feel you cannot survive, you can.
- The intense feelings of grief can be overwhelming and frightening. This is normal. You are not going crazy; you are grieving.
- You may experience feelings of guilt, confusion, and anger, even fear. These are all common responses to grief.
- You may even have thoughts of suicide. This, too, is common. It does not mean you will act on those thoughts.
- Forgetfulness is a common, but temporary side effect. Grieving takes so much energy that other things will fade in importance.
- Keep asking "why" until you no longer need to ask.

- Healing takes time. Allow yourself the time you need to grieve.
- Grief has no predictable pattern or timetable. Though there are elements of commonality in grief, each person and each situation is unique.
- If you can delay making major decisions, do so.
- The path of grief is one of twists and turns and you may often feel you are getting nowhere. Remember that even setbacks are a kind of progress.
- This is the hardest thing you will ever do. Be patient with yourself.
- Seek out people who are willing to listen when you need to talk and who understand you need to be silent.
- Give yourself permission to seek professional help.
- Avoid people who try to tell you what to feel and how to feel it and, in particular, those who think you should "be over it by now."
- Find a support group for survivors that provides a safe place for you to express your feelings or simply a place to go to be with other survivors who are experiencing some of the same things you are going through.

Explaining Suicide to a Child

"What should I tell the children?" A question often asked after the suicide of a loved one.

The answer—**the truth**.

Many people still believe it is best to shield children from the truth, that somehow this will protect them. More often than not, the opposite is true. Misleading children, evading the truth, or telling falsehoods to them about how someone died can do much more harm than good; if they happen to hear the truth from someone else, their trust in you can be difficult to regain. Not knowing can be terrifying and hurtful. We've always been told that "honesty is the best policy" and just because the subject is suicide, that doesn't mean this time is any different.

What children might be feeling after losing someone they love to suicide:

1. Abandoned—that the person who died didn't love them.
2. Feel the death is their fault—if they would have loved the person more or behaved differently.
3. Afraid that they will die too.
4. Worried that someone else they love will die or worry about who will take care of them.
5. Guilt—because they wished or thought of the person's death.
6. Sad.
7. Embarrassed—to see other people or to go back to school.
8. Confused.
9. Angry—with the person who died, at God, at everyone.
10. Lonely.
11. Denial—pretend like nothing happened.
12. Numb—can't feel anything.
13. Wish it would all just go away.

Chapter 55

Wounds

BUMPS AND BRUISES

Bruises, everyone gets them. Those ugly discolored patches that appear after you do something like slamming your elbow into the wall behind you, or taking a trip over your feet and falling hard. A bruise is caused by the damaging or breaking of a blood vessel, because of a blow to the skin. Some people bruise more easily than others. Children, for example, bruise much less easily than an elderly person would. Medications that interfere with blood clotting also help people to bruise more easily. Warfarin, a drug often prescribed to prevent clotting in those who have had clots in the legs or heart, can cause people to bruise severely.

Why Do Bruises Change Color?

Bruises are fairly predictable, you can often tell how old they are just by looking at them. When they first appear they will be reddish, a reflection of the blood trapped in the skin. After 1-2 days the bruise will appear blue or purple. By day 6 or so the bruise will be green and around days 8-9 it will be a yellowish brown. Usually the bruised area will look normal within 2-3 weeks.

What if it Doesn't Get Better or it Stays Swollen?

Sometimes this happens. If the bruise becomes firm and actually seems to become larger two things may have led to this. First of all, when the blood vessel broke, if it was a large amount of blood the body might have decided just to wall it off, rather than clean it up. This bump is called a hematoma, and it may need to be drained by your doctor.

A second problem, which is much less common, is when the body deposits calcium in the area of the injury. This area then becomes tender and firm and requires x-rays and a trip to the doctor. This condition is called heterotopic ossification.

Other Kinds of Bruises

Petechiae are little (3-3 millimeters) red dots that appear anywhere on the body, although the legs are most common. They are tiny little accumulations of blood. Often there are few of them and they usually indicate some sort of serious health problem.

Bruising around the belly button could be a result of bleeding in the abdomen.

Bruising behind the ear can indicate a skull fracture.

And lastly bruises that are raised, firm, and occur without any injury may be signs of a "autoimmune" disease, in which the body attacks it's own blood vessels. Your doctor should evaluate all of these sorts of bruises.

How to Treat Bruises

When bruising first occurs you can minimize the effects by using a cold compress. Place the ice in a bag or towel, as placing ice directly to the skin can cause frostbite. The cold reduces the flow of blood to the area and therefore reduces the size of the bruise. It also decreases the inflammation in the area and decreases swelling. If possible elevate the area to slow the blood flow. The lower the area is in relation to the heart the larger the bruise can be. Applying pressure also helps reduce blood flow and swelling. Another thing is to avoid medications that make it easier to bruise, however it is vital that you consult your doctor before making any changes to the medications you're on.

Cuts and Scrapes

How Do I Care For Cuts and Scrapes?

With all cuts and scrapes the most important thing to do first is to clean out the wound. Make sure you wash your hands before cleaning a wound to avoid transferring more dirt to the cut. Always wipe away from the wound when removing dirt and other particles that may be in the wound. When washing the wound use soap and water, but do not scrub because that may do more damage. *Hydrogen peroxide may be used but it is no substitute for soap and water!* Also in some cases iodine and hydrogen peroxide will delay healing. After the wound has been thoroughly washed look at it and determine how bad it is bleeding. Apply direct pressure with a clean dry cloth or sterile gauze bandage, while elevating limb (if possible) above the heart. This will slow bleeding and help a clot to form. If bleeding is spurting out of wound or bleeding continues heavily after pressure has been applied for 5-10 minutes stitches may be needed, so go to the hospital and have the wound checked out by your doctor as soon as possible. If the bleeding slows however cover the wound with a clean bandage. You may wish to apply a thin layer of antibacterial ointment to the wound first, to protect against infection. If the wounds are on the hands or feet avoid using these ointments after the first day. Make sure the wound is kept clean and dry while it heals. It is good to clean the wound and apply fresh bandages daily. To keep smiles on faces of those young and old try some of Crackles' funky bandages in zebra, rainbow, smiley faces, dinosaur and more!

Ointments

- Chose your ointment carefully. Some ointments like Bacitracin and Neo-mycin are common and best suited for small or minor cuts. If a large area is affected or if it is a more severe cut consult your doctor before using any ointments. It is advised to call your doctor if you have any ointment questions.
- If wound has not been properly cleaned the ointment may seal in bacteria. Another thing to be wary of is using too much ointment. If to much is applied it can increase the chance of infection, as bacteria is attracted to moisture. Apply only a thin layer to ensure the best protection.
- Always apply the ointment with a clean swab or gauze. Applying ointment from the tube may contaminate the tube and put future wounds at risk.
- Ointments may be used up to three times daily, but it is not very commonly recommended. Overuse of ointments may cause allergic reactions and will delay healing. Make sure to wash the wound before applying fresh ointment.

Who Should Always Go To The Doctor for Minor Wounds?

Diabetics and people who either have a long-term illness or are taking drugs that suppress the immune system should always go to the doctor, as they are in a more fragile state and are at greater risk of getting an infection.

What are Signs of Infection?

If the wound begins to drain greenish fluid, or is the skin around the wound is red, swollen and increasingly painful. Signs of an infection, known as Lymphangitis, is any red streaking on the skin around the wound may indicate an infection where fluid is draining from the tissues in the lymph system. This can be serious especially is accompanied by a fever. If signs of this infection are seen, get to the doctors as soon as possible.

Taking proper care of a wound by keeping it clean and covered can often prevent infection. Airtight bandages are recommended over "breathable" bandages. When applying fresh bandages make sure your hands are clean and the bandage remains sterile. It is advised that the bandage is opened over the wound and that the pad remains untouched except by the wound.

If wounds are neglected the following signs mean trouble:

- Redness, swelling, increased warmth and tenderness around the wound
- A strong or displeasing odor
- Chills and or fever
- The red streaking of lymphangitis
- Pus or watery discharge coming from the wound or collected beneath the skin around the wound.

Classification of Wounds

Incision: These cuts are often the result of some sharp object such as broken glass, knives and sharp edges. The amount of bleeding varies on the depth and extension of the cut. Some of these wounds require stitches.

Laceration: These are jagged irregularly shaped cuts or tears in the skin. Most lacerations are serous and require stitches, because of heavy bleeding. Chances of infection depend on the size, cause, and depth of the laceration. If the laceration seems severe, it should be seen and treated by a doctor. In these cases cover the wound with a clean cloth or sterile covering and seek medical treatment as soon as possible.

Punctures: Puncture wounds are caused by an object piercing the skin. These wounds range from minor to severe and should often be looked at by a doctor. The cause of a puncture wound is important, for example, if a rusted nail causes the wound the risk of infection is high and a tetanus shot may be needed. Splinters, glass, nails, pins, and other objects can also cause these wounds. Because the wound penetrates the skin (and in some cases, several layers of skin) they are often difficult to clean and infections are common.

In some cases, the puncture wound is very deep, such as a nail puncturing the foot. At times, the nail or other object may puncture the bone and introduce bacteria. These wounds are often marked by having difficulty removing the object from the affected area. If bone puncture is suspected, visit your doctor as soon as possible.

In more minor puncture wounds infection is not as common, but if redness and swelling persist, contact your doctor.

What About Those Tetanus Shots?

Most people (in the U.S.) have been immunized against this bacteria. If it has been five years since you received your last booster shot, and you get a puncture wound, you should get another to protect against tetanus infection. If you've never had a tetanus shot, or you have had fewer than three shots you may need to take a medication known as Tetanus Immunoglobulin to prevent the infection of this bacteria.

Severe Bleeding Injuries

1. Lay the person down. If possible, position the person's head slightly lower than the trunk, or elevate the legs. This position reduces the chances of fainting by increasing blood flow to the brain. If possible, elevate the site of bleeding.
2. Remove any obvious debris or dirt from the wound. Do not remove any objects pierced

into the victim. Do not probe the wound or attempt to clean it at this point. Your principal concern is to stop the loss of blood.

3. Apply pressure directly on the wound with a sterile bandage, clean cloth or even a piece of clothing. If nothing else is available, use your hand.
4. Maintain pressure until the bleeding stops. When it does, bind the wound tightly with adhesive tape or a bandage. If none is available, use a piece of clean clothing.
5. If the bleeding continues and seeps through the gauze or other material you are holding on the wound, do not remove it. Instead, add more absorbent material on top of it.
6. If the bleeding does not stop with direct pressure, you may need to apply pressure to the major artery that delivers blood to the area of the wound. In the case of a wound on the hand or lower arm, for example, squeeze the main artery in the upper arm against the bone. Keep your fingers flat; with the other hand, continue to exert pressure on the wound itself.
7. Immobilize the injured body part once the bleeding has been stopped. Leave the bandages in place and get the injured person to the emergency room as soon as possible.